Q MindFit Mastery™
Catalog

Q MindFit Product Resources
Table Of Contents

Q Exclusives

GoPro with Q MindFit Series 4

Achievement & Performance

iCan 5

Life Mastery Series 7

Sales Mastery Series 10

Behavior/Recovery

Alcohol-Free Series 12

Freedom From Addiction Series 14

Healing Meditations For Abuse Survivors 16

PTSD Recovery Series 18

Smoking Cessation Series 20

Children

Autism - The Children's Opportunity for Brilliance 22

Enlightened Children Series 24

Optimizing Your Children's Inner Potential 26

Health

Diabetes (Type I) Active Lifestyle Plan 28

Freedom from Irritable Bowel Syndrome 30

Gluten-Free Lifestyles 31

Heart Healthy Lifestyles 33

Healthy Sleeping Habits Series 36

Natural Lyme Relief Breakthrough 37

Mind Over Menopause 39

Pain-Free Lifestyle Series 41

Stress-Free Childbirth 43

Stress-Free Dentistry Series 45

Vibrant Health Series 46

Learning
Accelerated Learning Series   48

Lifestyle
Better Life Me   50
Blue Sky – Pro. Airline Series   52
Brain Fitness Series   54
Finding Love & Building Winning Relationships   56
Life-Mastery Series   58
Stress Reduction   60

Quick Start & AM/PM Series
10 Min AM Sessions   61
20 Min PM Sessions   61

Sports/Athletic Performance
Blue Chip Basketball   62
Mental Coaching For Golf   63
SportZone™ Series   65

Wealth
Wealth Consciousness Series   67

Weight Loss
Habits of Naturally Thin People   69

Q Sciences Products
EMPowerplus™ Q96   76
Cellerciser   77

What the media has to say about Q MindFit Technology   78
What the research has to say about Frequency Following Response   79
Q MindFit   85
Books Featuring Q MindFit Technology   88

THE QMindFit EXPERIENCE

PERSONAL ACHIEVEMENT HAS COME INTO THE LIGHT!

In just 20 relaxing minutes—the average time for a full Q MindFit session—you can unwind, decompress, undo the damaging effects of chronic daily stress, reduce or eliminate tension and worry, and retrain your brain for optimum performance and quality sleep.

Not only that, regular use can boost your energy, improve your attitude, inspire a healthy lifestyle, get rid of bad habits, instill new positive behaviors, and improve quality of life…all of which will make you a hero amongst your family and friends.

And the best part? Q MindFit can now help you supercharge your attitude and transform old thinking into the actions you need to build a thriving Q Sciences business.

The sessions below are specially designed by brain entrainment expert Dr. Patrick Porter (PhD) to help you reach the deepest levels of relaxation, where super-learning happens naturally. Then, at that optimized level of mind, you can rehearse the habits and patterns of the world's most successful network marketers and make them your own!

QS01-Q Sciences Experience 15 Mins

Dr. Porter has taken the stress out of explaining the Q MindFit technology to new members and prospects. What better way for your prospects to learn all about the science and benefits of Q MindFit than through a direct experience with the top expert in the field, Dr. Patrick Porter, as their guide?

QS02-Developing Your Why

What gets your juices flowing? Dr. Porter will help you explore—at the other-than-conscious level—the true motivation behind your actions. Your WHY is the fuel that will motivate you in both good and bad times. With this inner focus on your values and beliefs, you will build a valuable organization you can be proud to call your own.

QS03-Sharing Q Sciences with Passion & Confidence

Whether motivating retail customers to take back the power of their health or motivating your team, it all starts with your passion and confidence. You will explore mental techniques to help you ramp up your confidence and make your passion shine, making you the go-to person in your community for the life-changing Q Sciences product line.

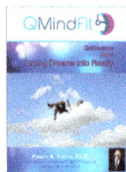

QS04-Turning Dreams Into Reality

Whether your dream is to help a family member or friend with the Q Sciences products or to build an international organization, it all starts with action steps. You will use a time-tested technique for building timelines to turn your dreams into reality. You will create a life of choice instead of a life of chance. Take the guesswork out of your future by creating the life of your dreams today.

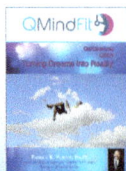

QS05-Going PRO with Q Sciences

We all know of a special someone who seems to have a magical ability to build a booming business. With the new science of Q MindFit, you can learn the technique of modeling excellence, which will have you absorbing the skills of business masters as if by osmosis. You'll step on the fast track to success by thinking and acting like a consummate business pro!

QS06-Playing the Prospecting Game

Success starts by interacting with life as a game, so you can have fun while you're succeeding. You will learn the techniques that transform the fear of asking for business into the joy of playing the game of prospecting. You will realize that you have been given a mission to share Q Sciences with the world.

QS07-Your Team Building Game Plan

Q Sciences has afforded you a wonderful opportunity. You get to choose the team that supports your dreams and goals. Dr. Porter will guide you through a proven process for building a mastermind group as described in Napoleon Hill's book, *Think and Grow Rich*. This mastermind team is your source of inspiration that will fuel your Q Sciences business.

Creator of the Q MindFit

Dr. Patrick Porter has been on the cutting edge of brainwave entrainment for 28 years. He is the author of 8 personal development books and over 500+ Self-Mastery Technology audio recordings, including these Q eXclusives!

Empower your business with QMindFit

QSciences.com

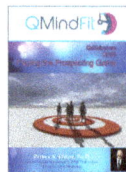

I Can. Therefore, I Will
The Definitive Guide to Sculpting Your Destiny

Based on the work of Carolyn Hansen, Dr. Patrick Porter (PhD) has designed a Brainwave Entrainment (BWE) series that will help you to super-charge the core message in 'I Can, Therefore I Will'. Available online at self-masterytechnology.com

These sessions are designed to train the subconscious to work in harmony with your conscious mind as you read through and practice the core message in this course.

Below, you will find in detail what each audio CD will teach you:

iCan01 – Building Your New Thought Generator

New thoughts lead to new actions. In this program Dr. Porter will help you through the science of Neuro-Linguistic Programming (NLP) to use your most powerful asset, "Your Mind." As you learn that thoughts are more powerful than things and thoughts create things you will begin to think beyond the past in new and better ways that will help you create the life you really want.

iCan02 – Beyond Positive Thinking

In Dr. Porter's over 27 years of helping people he has seen the 'flaws' of positive thinking alone and how it actually prevents people from taking action. With this work Carolyn has distilled down the secrets to moving beyond positive thinking into a world of infinite possibilities where your other-than-conscious can take over and put your success on autopilot.

iCan03 – Change Your Inner Self Talk – Change Your Life

We have constant conversations within ourselves. Is yours supportive and positive or demotivating and negative? Self-talk is the lubrication to action. With the right inner talk powerful action can take place. In this program Dr. Porter guides you through Carolyn's breakthrough exercises that will having you making your positive change in days instead of months.

iCan04 – Taking the 1st Step to Your – 'I Can' Action

All behaviors are useful in the right context. The problem is if the subconscious is left up to its programming, it will continue to give you what you have already got. Dr. Porter will teach you how to transform negative behaviors into positive patterns of improvement. Imagine your life when procrastination leads to motivation and when fear transforms into personal power.

Achievement & Performance

iCan05 – Creating Your 'I Can' – Challenge Breakthroughs

During Carolyn's years of research she has noticed that there is a strong desire for a challenge. With this program Dr. Porter will show you why it is important to face these challenges and plan for success instead of counting on failure. Today is the day you choose to succeed knowing that how you do the smallest of things you do the big things.

iCan06 – Living The Dream...Infinite – Possibilities & Opportunities

Reading and assimilating the wisdom found in the "I Can. Therefore I Will" is the first step. With this breakthrough session you will employ your access to an infinite mind. Dr. Porter will teach you the time tested techniques used by the world's greatest inventors to awaken their genius in their dreams. As you harness the power of your dreams you will achieve the seemingly impossible by accessing your inventive mind through the use of neuro-sensory algorithms to awaken your dreams.

This course consists of 8 components:

Carolyn Hansen's The Definitive Guide Of 'I Can. Therefore I Will'

The Goal Setting Work Book
Building Your New Thought Generator MP3 Audio
Beyond Positive Thinking MP3 Audio
Change Your Inner Self Talk – Change Your Life MP3 Audio
Taking the 1st Step to Your – 'I Can' Action Plan MP3 Audio
Creating Your 'I Can' – Challenge breakthroughs MP3 Audio
Living The Dream...Infinite – Possibilities & Opportunities MP3 Audio

As you devour the content here, it will reveal the secrets behind creating your dream life.

The Goal Setting Work Book

This goal setting workbook is very important because we will break down the most difficult parts about goal setting into easy baby steps. It will keep you accountable to your word and help you to internalize daily action habits so that your habits will become a permanent part of your life.

Here's what you'll discover in this workbook: (available online)

Exercises on what you did great last year and how to propel this year

Set an intention to increase your focus on certain areas of attention

Resolve to change certain bad habits and take on good ones

Set definite goals and propel your success

Harness the power of specificity

How to set goals from your heart so you will succeed at all costs

How to break them all down into baby steps so everything is achievable and more...

Life Mastery Series
Patrick K. Porter, Ph.D.

Throughout your life, from parents, teachers, and society, you were taught what to think. With the breakthrough processes of creative visualization and relaxation, you are going to discover how to think. With this knowledge you will literally become a software engineer for your own mind. On the Life-Mastery journey, you will explore the processes that best suit your needs for creating limitless personal improvement and success in your life.

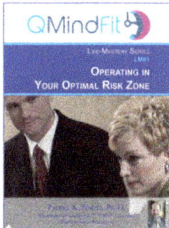

LM01 – Operating in Your Optimal Risk Zone

The startling truth is, all human beings must have risk in their lives to thrive and feel fulfilled. Listen to this session and you'll know how to leverage risk for personal advancement and easily accomplish your loftiest goals. The dot com bust turned risk into a four letter word. Yet executives and companies that don't employ risk can face extinction. In creating the Optimal Risk Zone, Dr. Patrick Porter researched the mindset of the controlled risk-takers who launched the high-tech industry. Then, using CVR, those thoughts and behaviors can be virtually downloaded into your mind.

LM02 – Ask, Believe & Receive Visualization

The universe operates on specific laws. These *invisible* laws are always *manifesting* your physical reality. The universe never *tries* anything; it only *does*. This visualization calls upon the *Law of Attraction*, and helps you to become a conscious creator. You will discover how you designed, at the core of your being, to be an active participant in the enfoldment of your relationships, wealth and happiness. Now, without even trying or having to struggle, success will come as naturally as the sun rises and sets. Imagine how much easier your life can become when you are in perfect harmony with universal law!

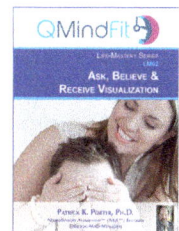

LM03 – The Secret Power of Self-talk

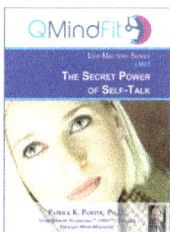

On average, you give yourself over 5,000 messages a day. With this process you will discover how to weed your mental garden of negative thoughts and to sow new, more positive thoughts. You will use the same four-step process that has helped thousands of people neutralize fear, anxiety and worry. Using CVR, you discover the secret power of self-talk to easily create the habits, patterns, and beliefs that can put your success on autopilot.

LM04 – Activate the Magnetic Power of Your Dreams

Many of the great inventors of the past discovered that your dreams are a powerful way to communicate with your other-than-conscious mind. You will unlock the most powerful computer on earth as you discover creative ways to use your dreams to visualize solutions to everyday problems. Get ready to step out of the past and into a bright and compelling future!

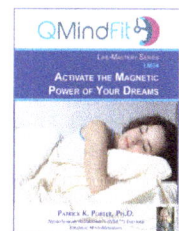

LM05 – Become A Personal Success Magnet

With this CVR process, Dr. Patrick Porter will guide you through powerful and easy techniques for attracting success into your life. Your new thoughts will act as a magnet that draws the right people and opportunities to you, and guides you in making the right decisions. Sit back and relax in the laboratory of your mind as you tap into your other-than-conscious storehouse of success-breeding thoughts—the thoughts that will draw success to you as naturally as you draw your next breath.

Achievement & Performance

LM06 – Whole Brain Motivation & Unending Drive

During this CVR journey, you will discover new ways of tapping into the creative right side of your brain. Then, using the left logical side of the brain, you will create a timeline for success. When you harness the power of whole brain thinking, you can accomplish even the most difficult tasks with ease. The balanced success that others only dream of will be yours as you master this visualization.

LM07 – Step On The Fast Track To Personal Success

Sir Isaac Newton once said that if he had achieved anything with his work, such as his laws of motion and gravity, it was "by standing on the shoulders of giants." With this process, you will explore what I call *The Picasso Factor* and find out why it was easy for Gandhi, Einstein and other masters to put their success on autopilot. By using the principle of mentoring found in this visualization, you will tap into your own inner genius and be on the fast track to success. What is *The Picasso Factor*? You'll have to listen to find out!

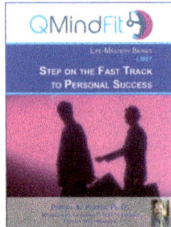

LM08 – Enthusiasm, Focus & Flexibility…
Your Keys To Success

Imagine the improvements you can make in your life once you activate the powerful storehouse of your other-than-conscious mind that will give you all the enthusiasm, focus and flexibility you need on a day-to-day basis. During this visualization, Dr. Patrick Porter will guide you to find your own internal success coach, who will take you step-by-step in the direction of your goals. With this mental exercise you will easily manifest your dreams into reality.

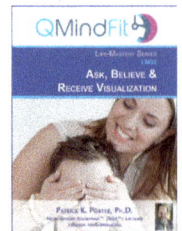

LM09 – Harness The Power Of Change

You will discover why *change*, the only constant in the universe, can be your most powerful ally. When you let go of the fear of change, and harness its power instead, you are tapping into the most potent force in the universe. When you try new things in the laboratory of your mind, you erase fear and embrace the action steps necessary to maximize your results.

LM10 – Awaken Your Senses and Create Your Future

Your senses can be likened to the keyboard on a computer. Through sight, sound, touch, smell and taste, your brain takes in information from the world around you. Now you can learn to use your senses to magnetize success into your life. It becomes simple to be the person you were destined to be when you create change at the other-than-conscious level of your mind. It's literally as easy as seeing, hearing, feeling and maybe even tasting or smelling the future of your dreams.

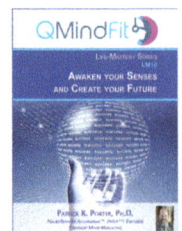

LM11 – Power Phrases For Powerful Actions

Discover how affirmative words and phrases can create a powerful mental image of a healthy, wealthy and vibrant new you. You will notice how these positive affirmations let your other-than-conscious mind quickly put into motion all the right actions at the right time to lead you to a life filled with the results you really want.

LM12 – Eliminate Negative Thinking and Harness The Power of Optimism

You can't help but be bombarded with negative thoughts and beliefs; it's on the radio, television and in the newspaper. With this powerful process, Dr. Patrick Porter will guide you into altered states, where you'll discover ways of breaking through to your creative optimistic mind. Once there you will be visualizing solutions to your life challenges. Imagine what you will create in your life as you eliminate the negative and let the flow of optimistic thinking create instantaneous solutions.

LM13 – Transform Procrastination into Total Motivation

All behaviors are useful in the right context. During this CVR process, Dr. Porter will guide you through a seven-step transformation process that will end procrastination and convert that energy into the usable motivation you'll need to complete tasks, start new projects, or live the healthy lifestyle you always dreamed of. Using the power of possibility has never been easier as you relax and realize your goals.

LM14 – Journey to the Creativity Zone

In today's stress-filled, hectic world it is often difficult to quiet your mind enough to tap into your innate creativity. Yet, for many of us, creativity is essential to our work performance. And, for all of us, it is vital for leading a balanced life. As you kick back and relax, Dr. Porter guides to a mind state where you can enhance any creative endeavor. This session is truly an inner journey to the place in your mind where ideas abound and solutions are readily available.

Sales Mastery Series
Patrick K. Porter, Ph.D.

Discover the powerful selling methods of sales masters! When you use this amazing series, you'll build your self-confidence, master your time, and learn to overcome all objections. Visualize and realize your brighter sales future today.

SM01 – Sales Confidence through Self-Confidence

To have confidence in your sales skills, you need confidence in yourself. In this dynamic session, Dr. Patrick Porter will show you how to generate resources you never knew you had. Take control of your own self-confidence in order to organize your thoughts, put priorities in place and take control of your sales… and your life!

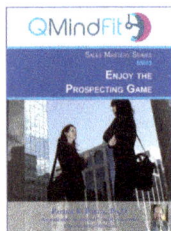

SM02 – Supercharge Your Sales Skills

You already have all the abilities you need to become a sales superstar. This exciting process will help you organize those resources to eliminate cold-call reluctance and discover the secrets known by true sales pros. Sit back, relax, and find out how to supercharge your sales skills!

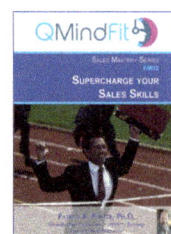

SM03 – Enjoying the Prospecting Game

All sales masters know networking is the key to finding a need and helping prospects fill it. This refreshing process by Dr. Patrick Porter teaches you to develop your infinite referral system and make all the money you desire. When you approach sales with the mindset of a child, prospecting is not only easy… it's fun!

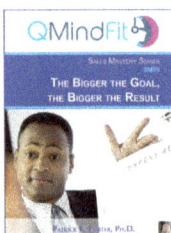

SM04 – Creating Your Sales Success Plan

Use this enjoyable and effortless process to discover quick, easy steps for implementing and working your personal success plan. When you have a plan, you create unlimited success in your sales career, as well as a balanced life at home. It's fun to master your career and your life!

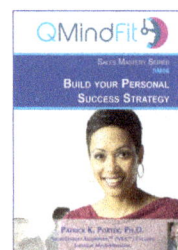

SM05 – The Bigger the Goal, the Better the Result

Sit back and relax as Dr. Patrick Porter shows you how to eliminate small thinking from your sales and your life. Break the chains of old, conscious thought and use your creative mind to create bigger goals and better results. Expand your ability to be flexible around the most difficult people and use quick techniques for closing the sale with even the most negative person.

SM06 – Build Your Personal Success Strategy

Creating balance in your life is easy when you use your other-than-conscious. With this revitalizing process, you'll quickly wipe out procrastination and energize your daily sales activities. Discover your dynamic self-image that's been waiting to shine. When you activate your creative genius, your possibilities are endless!

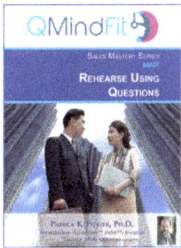

SM07 – Rehearse Using Questions to Understand Your Prospect's Business

Enter the theater of your mind, where you visualize and realize your sales goals! Discover the ease of working through success scripts—and see the unbelievable results play out before you—to easily overcome potential objections. When you know the criteria your prospect uses to make decisions, it's a snap to identify additional advantages to using your product or service. This process shows you that you plan to succeed when you leave nothing to chance.

SM08 – Fill the Need, Close the Sale

Follow along as Dr. Patrick Porter shows you how to use this unique questioning approach. You'll learn to quickly break the trust barrier and discover your prospect's needs. Once you know your prospect's needs and values, closing the sale is as easy as taking a breath of fresh air!

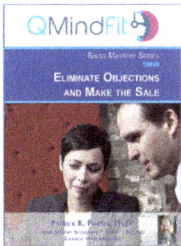

SM09 – Eliminate Objections and Make the Sale

Your greatest sales obstacle lies in the mind of your prospect. This creative visualization process trains your brain to listen for and overcome objections—before your prospects know they have them! Selling is easy when you use the simple laws of persuasion.

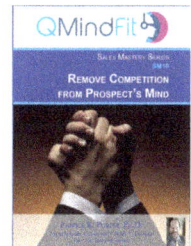

SM10 – Remove Your Competition from the Mind of Your Prospect

Your prospect has many options in the marketplace, and your job is to show them you're the best choice. Now, you can get your prospect to eliminate your competition from contention—without you using a single negative word against them. It's easier than you think when you use these four simple steps!

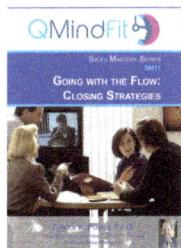

SM11 – Going with the Flow: Closing Strategies & Objection Prevention

This refreshing process by Dr. Patrick Porter allows you to remove the stress of closing the deal. Objections are part of the sales game, but you'll learn how the power of "no" can actually help you reach your sales goals. By using this simple three-step process, you'll be ready and able to close the most difficult prospect. Master your mental state, and you'll master any sales situation.

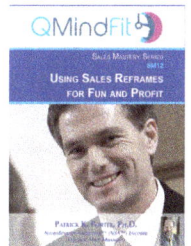

SM12 – Using Sales Reframes for Fun & Profit

Learn how to transition, or reframe, a negative statement into a positive one with this motivating session. Even the most difficult sale is easy when you can turn resistance into cooperation. Master the pre-frame and reframe and you'll help your prospects sell themselves!

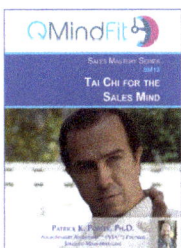

SM13 – Tai Chi for the Sales Mind

Harmony is one of the most powerful forces in the universe. Your own negative thoughts work against you and harmfully affect your sales performance. When you use this inspirational technique, you will elevate your thoughts to the highest level without stress or struggle. When your mind is on your side, anything is possible!

Freedom From Alcohol
Patrick K. Porter, Ph.D.

Patrick Porter, PhD is the creator of Hidden Solutions, a program offered by the Arizona Health Council to help D.U.I. offenders reclaim their lives. Now you can learn the hidden solutions that reside within you—solutions that can free you from your desire for alcohol for good. You'll learn to transform your alcohol addiction into something far more positive—an addiction to a healthy, balanced lifestyle. All you'll need to do is relax with these processes, which are based on Dr. Porter's personal experiences with his own addictive family and the twelve-step method that helped them heal. You'll quickly discover that the life you desire is within reach once you take control of your future—once you tune into the unlimited power that is far greater than your conscious mind.

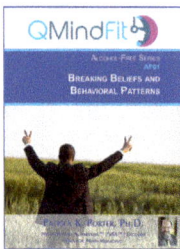

AF01 – Breaking Beliefs and Behavioral Patterns
Alcohol is a killer addiction that is often at the core of many psychological, emotional and relationship problems. In this CVR session, Dr. Porter will guide you in evaluating the problem from the creative right side of your brain where new options can be realized and implemented. Then, with mental rehearsal, your logical left brain will show you how to use these solutions in your every day life.

AF02 – Reclaiming Your Power
The first step in AA is to admit that you are powerless over alcohol and that your life has become unmanageable. Now that you have chosen to be alcohol free, it's time to retrain your brain, which is a goal-striving organism that needs direction. You will achieve your goal by building your plan and then planning to succeed. By using this dynamic CVR process as a step-by-step guide, you will allow your other-than-conscious mind to guide you into a life where alcohol has no claim on you.

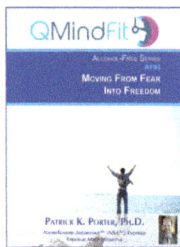

AF03 – Moving From Fear into Freedom
Every successful recovery starts with the belief that a power greater than one's conscious mind can restore sanity. As you learn to trust in this guiding force, you will release the fear and frustration of the past. From there, it becomes easy to take back your power and create a healthy lifestyle free from alcohol.

AF04 – Using the Power of Intention for a Healthy Life
Now that you have made the decision to turn your will and your life over to the care of your other-than-conscious mind, you can rid yourself of the behaviors of the past and step into the alcohol-free life you were born to live. You will discover ways to de-stress, re-focus, and enjoy life more fully each day, one day at a time.

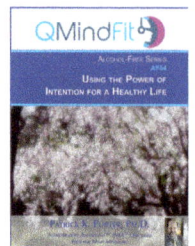

AF05 – Tuning Into the Power of Change
It has been said that those who do not learn from the past are doomed to relive it. In this process you will admit to yourself (and to other human beings) the exact nature of your wrongs. Since the brain doesn't know the difference between real or imagined, you can take this difficult step toward forgiving yourself—a step that will ultimately free you from the guilt of past behaviors.

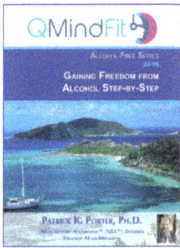

AF06 – Gaining Freedom from Alcohol Step by Step

In previous processes you made a fearless moral inventory of yourself and your life. Now it's time to take a safe and easy step-by-step approach to freeing yourself from alcohol. The truth is that you are more capable than you think. It's now time to eliminate any negative thinking that may be keeping you tied to the debilitating effects of alcohol. Learn to forgive, forget, and move on with this unique healing process.

AF07 – Living Life Alcohol Free

Now that you have developed a powerful new mindset, you are ready to have any defects of character removed. Imagine the freedom, self-confidence, and success you will experience now that you have conquered the alcoholic behaviors of the past. Mentally rehearse living the rest of your life in health, wealth, and vitality with this calming process. It all starts with a commitment to living your life from the highest moral ground.

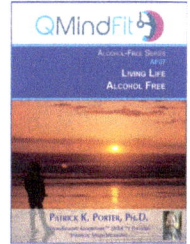

AF08 – Rebuilding Your Life

By now you have likely realized that you have always done your best given the limited knowledge you had available. The good news is, while going through this CVR series, you have been slowly and humbly removing your shortcomings. Now that you have discovered the freedom of choice, you will use this process to come to the conclusion that leading an alcohol free life will be good for you and your family. How wonderful for you to now walk tall and proud without ever again using alcohol as a crutch!

AF09 – Taking Responsibility

Use CVR to take control now so you can achieve the life of your dreams. You have within you untapped talent and skills that you have yet to realize. Dr. Porter gently guides you through this healing process of visualizing all people you have harmed, and making amends to them all. You will do this first in your mind and then, if appropriate, in the physical world.

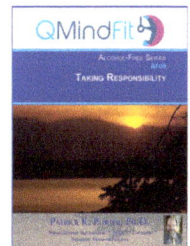

AF10 – Eliminating Negative Self-Talk

You might not be able to make direct amends to all the people you have hurt; however, you can rid yourself of those harmful behaviors and step into the alcohol-free life you were born to live. Learn to de-stress, re-focus, and enjoy life more fully each day while you leave the shame and guilt of the past in the past.

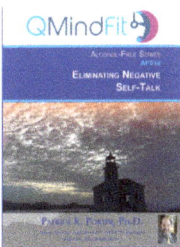

AF11 – Clean and Healthy and Loving It!

Once you've made it this far, imagine how great you will feel about yourself. One day at a time you will have finally, once and for all, conquered alcohol—an impossible task made possible once you found the will to take up the challenge. This is a time for celebrating the brand new mindset you've created—one that will keep you clean and sober even in the most difficult times.

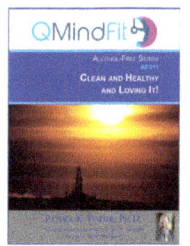

AF12 – Mind & Body Solutions Alcohol Free

As you work to create the mind-body connection of health and wellness, a deep inner knowing of your true self will develop, keeping you focused on the best outcomes for you, your body, and everyone concerned.

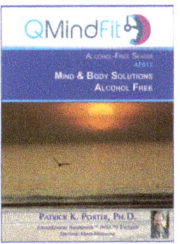

AF13 – Awakening to a New Reality

In this final process you will develop a deep desire for honesty along with the ability to take personal inventory and recognize when you are wrong. Now that you have had an awakening as the result of these processes, you will develop a lifelong desire to practice these principles in all your affairs. Now that you know that if the mind can conceive it, you can achieve it, the possibilities for our life are virtually limitless!

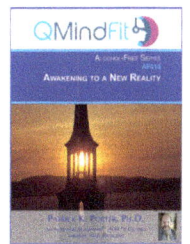

Freedom From Addiction
Patrick K. Porter, Ph.D.

Addiction comes in many forms, but the underlying cause remains the same. For every addiction there is an underlying positive intention that the mind is trying to fulfill. Now you can use the power of your mind—through creative visualization and relaxation (CVR)—to find more appropriate ways to satisfy that positive intention without the destructive behaviors of the past. Dr. Patrick Porter's ground-breaking CVR program for overcoming addiction can work for just about any addiction including the following:

Alcoholism - Anorexia - Bulimia - Codependency - Gambling - Marijuana Narcotics - Prescription Drugs - Overeating - Overspending - Pornography - Self-Injury

FA01 – Personal Responsibility
Working With Your Other-Than-Conscious Mind to Manage Your Life

Most people who struggle with addictions have, in reality, simply lost their power of choice. Dr. Patrick Porter (PhD) will help you discover why trying to force a change with willpower only perpetuates the problem and how visualization is what will lead you to realization and freedom. You will discover how, by tapping into the power of your mind, you can rebuild your confidence (even in uncertain times) and bring into your consciousness (with sufficient force) the appropriate memories and choices that will lead you to living an addiction-free life—which is your birthright.

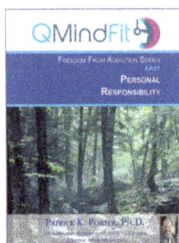

FA02 – Tapping Into a Power Greater Than You
to Restore Sanity to Your Life

With years of clinical experience, Dr. Patrick Porter has found that those who are willing to turn over their addiction to a greater power find the transition to addiction-free behavior easier, and they are far more likely to achieve lasting results. It has been repeatedly proven that, upon a simple cornerstone of faith, a spiritual structure of strength and resolve can be built. During this process, you will use your own concept of this *higher power* to reframe your past, and you will start today to live the life you were born to live.

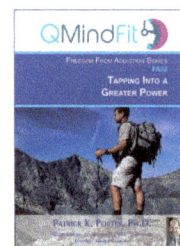

FA03 – Release Your Past and Embrace the Power of Change

In this process you will mentally make a decision to turn your will and your future over to the care of the creator, as you understand that creative force to be. During this visualization, you will release the bondage of the past so that this force for good may better do its will. By planning one day at a time, you will find that your challenges and stressors fall away as you create daily victories over them. Relax and bear witness to the flow of life, and it will help you tap into its power, love, and grace; your addiction-free new way of life will be the natural by-product.

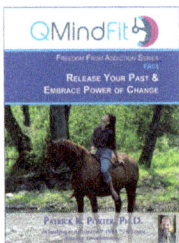

FA04 – Taking a Fearless Moral Inventory

Every behavior, even those that are negative, has a positive underlying intent. Dr. Patrick Porter will guide you through the process of discovering your positive intention and developing more appropriate ways of meeting it. You will experience a mental cleansing as you realize that, in the past, you did the very best you could with the information you had at the time. Today you will open to the truth about who you are and experience the release that comes when you forgive yourself. Once you search out your flaws, you can make a daily plan for avoiding what in the past caused your failure. You will soon be embracing your life free from addiction.

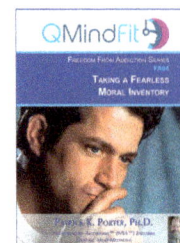

FA05 – Developing the Courage to Express and Release the Past

During this powerful visualization, you will gain the courage to express your regret to those you have wronged in the past. Even though this is perhaps the most difficult step, it is also the most liberating. No one likes to discuss defects with others; however, this is exactly what's needed to create the new state of balance in your life. This session will also take you through a visualization where you can communicate your request for forgiveness to those who are no longer in your life or are deceased. Dr. Porter will help you to rediscover the balance within yourself as you take this important step in the mental healing process.

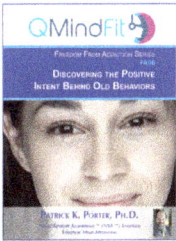

FA06 – Discovering the Positive Intent Behind Old Behaviors

It is human nature to stay attached to old habits even when those habits are no longer working. Fortunately, once you uncover the underlying positive intention behind the old behaviors, you can easily learn to meet those needs with new, more appropriate habits. Dr. Porter will guide you through this inner battle between old habits and new behaviors, and you will come out the other side with positive new insights. You will release the emotional pain of the past and create the balance essential to making changes in your life one day at a time.

FA07 – Humility—Your Key To Lasting Change

Cultivating humility, along with letting your greater power work in your life, is perhaps the least discussed in addiction recovery groups, yet it is probably the most potent as it relates to lasting life changes. Humility embodies the miracle of transformation, and all it takes is turning over to your higher power the old unhealthy thinking patterns. After all, it was your best thinking that brought you to where you are now. If your best thinking could have helped you out of this situation, it would have already happened. In this session, Dr. Porter will help you reframe the past, foster a positive mind-set, and mold the present into a healthy agent for change.

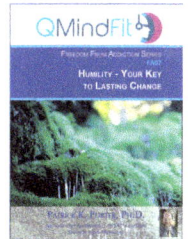

FA08 – Trying New Things for a New Beginning

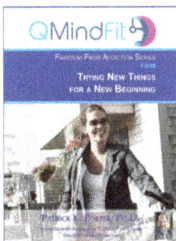

Tapping into the power of your other-than-conscious mind goes beyond doing what you have always done. To be liberated from the defeatist attitude of the past, you must embrace change and try new things. It has been said that if you are a craftsman with only a hammer, you will think everything is a nail. The key to lasting change is in having options. There is nothing wrong with persistence, but those who have created a life free from addiction have done so by developing new ways of thinking and acting. In this session, Dr. Patrick Porter will guide you through the resource organizer where you will discover skills you didn't even know you had.

FA09 – Social Housecleaning from the Inside Out

During this session you will visualize cleaning up all the bruised relationships and the pockets of guilt, pain, fear, resentment, and sadness that are stored inside, stuck to shameful past deeds. Dr. Porter will help you through this mental healing by guiding you to that power greater than yourself where you will release the past hurts that may be stopping you from loving other people and yourself. You will learn to trust in the guidance of your higher power right now, in the present.

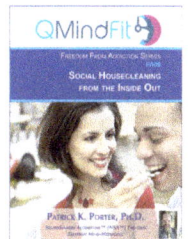

FA10 –Becoming a Bridge-Builder for More Positive Relationships

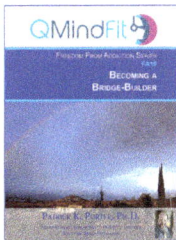

Being a bridge-builder means that cleaning up your past becomes a way of life. As you enter this working relationship with your other-than-conscious mind, Dr. Porter will guide you through your next step, which is to grow in understanding and effectiveness. This is no overnight matter; it will continue for the rest of your life, one day at a time. With this realization you will learn to be vigilant over the part of you that wants to hold on to selfishness, dishonesty, resentment, and fear. When these crop up, you will trust the power greater than yourself to remove them.

FA11 – Let Go and Go with the Flow (safe place)

In this process, you will create an internal compass to help you stay the course free from addiction. Dr. Porter will teach you techniques to keep you grounded in reality so that the old attitudes, behaviors, or beliefs that brought out the addictive behaviors stay at bay while new more appropriate behaviors are formed. You will learn to keep your options in a safe place by keeping conscious contact with that power that is greater than you.

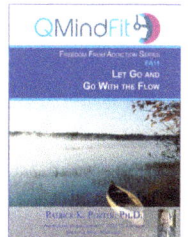

FA12 – Taking Care of Today by Planning a Bright Future

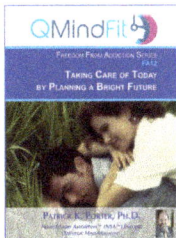

Dr. Porter will help you stay focused on the most important moment in time, NOW. By taking care of today and staying with a one-day-at-a-time philosophy, you can look forward to a bright and compelling future. This visualization will open you to unlimited possibilities as you make your mind available as a tool for sharing your recovery success on a daily basis.

FA13 – Staying Connected to Your Higher Power

The real secret to remaining free from addiction for a lifetime involves a spiritual awakening. When Dr. Porter did his research, he found that those who stayed connected to this infinite stream of intelligence stayed free from the addictions of the past and kept a fresh perspective on today. Problem solving takes on a new level of creativity when you are connected to this power greater than yourself. You will learn a simple technique that is already being used by thousands to stay connected. You will also be amazed by how simple it is when you trust in the process of change.

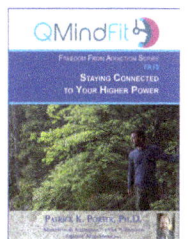

Healing Meditations for Child Abuse Survivors
Patrick K. Porter, Ph.D.
Inspired by the Reaching Out Child Abuse Monument

This series by Dr. Patrick Porter is inspired by Dr. Michael Irving's Reaching Out Child Abuse Monument. These visualizations will assist you in seeing yourself as a remarkable person who has the courage to live through adversity and rise above and beyond a kind of cruelty that never should have happened. You will see that you have a hopeful, problem-solving spirit with a commitment to make more of your life.

Your survival through adversity was heroic, which means you have all the power and resources you need to create a positive mind and a vibrant and enjoyable life. You will be encouraged to think comforting thoughts and to know the ways in which you are safe. These meditations will help you to recognize that the trauma occurred a long time ago. You now have the comfort of distance and the power to move forward. Listening will help you get grounded as you come to understand that a memory is not abuse; memories are thoughts, and feelings and are within your power to change. You can embrace the power of your inner wisdom. You can release the emotions of the past. You will realize that no matter what has happened, you get better and better every day, and you will find pleasure and comfort in the world you create. What you imagine is what you become.

HMS01 – Meditation on Hope and Healing
In this meditation, you will reflect on hope as your birthright and as one of the most powerful forces in the universe. You will let healing hope radiate through your spirit and will focus on thoughts that bring hope, comfort and calm. You will meditate on the people you can lean on for support and turn to for nurturing. You will contemplate thoughts that bring you hope, and that move you closer to comfort and calm. The hopes of your dreams are what you receive.

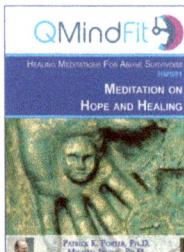

HMS02 – Meditation for Empowerment
During this meditation, you will reflect on your inner strengths and the empowerment that comes from believing in yourself. You will meditate on feelings associated with your important accomplishments and how others see your strengths. In acknowledging your empowerment and victories, you can come to trust your inner voice and intuition. You will dream big and know you can follow those dreams.

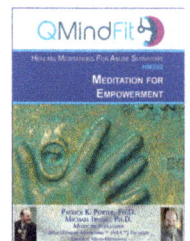

HMS03 – Meditation for Safety and Containment
This mediation will help you create safety and containment through visualizing a safe room. You will explore what you need for your individual safe room and create it as your perfect place of relaxation. You will also practice separation and distancing though a locked box or other container. This meditation is a celebration of the power, resiliency and amazement within your inner wisdom and other-than-conscious mind.

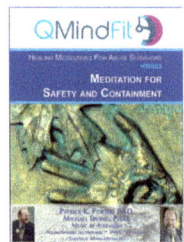

HMS04 – Meditation for Healing Shame
Abuse survivors often carry a heavy burden of shame and humiliation. This meditation will help you free yourself from these destructive and limiting feelings. It will assist you with internalizing the truth that the abuse was not your fault and that the shame does not belong to you. You will feel your power to release stuck patterns and beliefs of the past that no longer serve you. You will release shame and replace the emotion with joy and freedom.

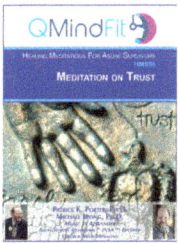

HMS05 – Meditation on Trust

Abuse robs the birthright of trust. Through this meditation, you will reawaken your innate ability to trust. You will explore what you need in your life and environment to feel safe and secure. Experiencing your "antennae" for trust and for mistrust will empower you. Safe, trusting people will fill your thoughts and begin to appear in your life.

HMS06 – Meditation on Self-Soothing

This meditation will support and nourish the positive and comforting feelings already inside of you so they will grow and blossom. You will practice breathing in calming energy and releasing stress as you become more relaxed and self-aware. Listening to this meditation will help you find more and more ways to self-sooth and nurture yourself.

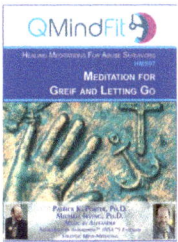

HMS07 – Meditation for Grief and Letting Go

This meditation will support you in moving through and beyond the grief associated with child abuse. You will acknowledge and accept the presence of grief and then give it permission to be resolved and released. The meditation will provide you the release and freedom that letting go of the past creates. You will then take that freedom with you into your present and future.

HMS08 Meditation for Healing the Inner Child

This meditation will assist you in connecting with the innocence of your inner child. You will assure your inner child that there is safety and benefit in healing and letting go. You will help your inner child make sense of the hurt from long ago so you can restore your feelings of worthiness and reclaim your ability to love and be loved.

HMS09 – Meditation on Celebrating Victory

This meditation will focus on celebrating the victory of having survived and thrived through the adversities of childhood and the challenging process of healing. You will reflect on the many ways you can be proud of yourself. Just to get through your childhood was an extraordinary achievement. Once you acknowledge this, your ability to embrace life today will be magnificent. You are a hero and your healing from adversity will make a difference in the lives of others.

HMS10 – Meditation to Heal Self-Blame

This meditation focuses on helping you to let go of self-blame and the guilt and destructive behaviors that frequently accompany a history of child abuse. You will focus on the reality that you did the best you could against insurmountable odds. This process will help you recognize that there is nothing wrong with you. As you release self-blame you will feel joy and freedom, and see yourself as a new you.

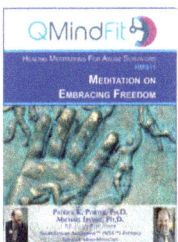

HMS11 – Meditation on Embracing Freedom

Through this meditation you will embrace and celebrate the freedom of having overcome the pain that lasted so long. You will celebrate your freedom and know the past is no longer a chain that binds you. This meditation will assist you with creating an ever-present force of freedom inside of you.

HMS12 – Meditation for Feeling Loved

This meditation focuses on reawakening your basic right to feel loved that was wounded by child abuse. You will reflect on times where you felt loved and notice where the "being loved" feeling is inside of you so you can let that feeling grow. You will meditate on attracting loving people to your life, knowing that what you see is what you create.

HMS13 – Safe Mountain Meadow Retreat

In this meditation you will create a safe mountain meadow retreat as an empowering inner sanctuary you can return to again and again. You will connect with the courage, bravery and life skills you have inside. You will experience your retreat as a protective place of containment and peacefulness. Your mountain meadow retreat will become a safe haven where you can go whenever you need to find refuge from troubling feelings or thoughts.

Breaking Through PTSD
with Neuro-Sensory Algorithms™

The Q MindFit Neuro-Sensory Algorithms (NSAs) audio system is uniquely designed to eliminate the symptoms of Post Traumatic Stress Disorder (PTSD). Through the combined neuro-training of NSAs and Strategic Mind Messaging™, the listener can learn to eliminate or cope with the emotions and anxiety resulting from a shocking, life-threatening, or otherwise highly unsafe experience. People who suffer from PTSD do so because they continue to re-experience the traumatic event or events in some way that affects them physically, mentally and emotionally. PTSD sufferers tend to avoid places, people, or other things that remind them of the event (avoidance), and are unusually sensitive to normal life experiences (hyper-arousal). Although this condition has likely existed since human beings have endured trauma, in the past such advanced brain training was not available, and standard clinical treatment can be a long process costing thousands of dollars. But now, with the help of the digital age and Q MindFit, results can be achieved affordably in the comfort of your own home. This technology will help you create the changes where they all started in the first place—your thinking. The Breaking Through PTSD series uses the most advanced patterns of Neuro-Linguistic Programming (NLP) to help you release the past, create balance in the present, and build a compelling future in which you are free of PTSD symptoms.

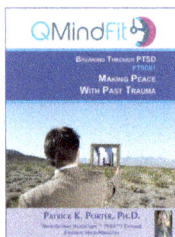

PTSD01 – Making Peace with Post Traumatic Stress Disorder
Dr. Patrick Porter (PhD) will help you resolve the inner conflict from past experiences. Armed with this new way of thinking, you will begin to rebuild your life in powerful new ways. Each session is designed to teach you a new way of thinking. While other programs tell you what to think, in this series you will learn how to think and why the best part of the past is over and how to move on to a new healing environment.

PTSD02 – Reclaim Your Future after PTSD
When trauma happens, it can feel as if your future has been destroyed by a single past experience. In this Strategic Mind Messaging session, Dr. Porter will help you build the resources you need so you not only survive but thrive in your new environment. We believe that every person has the resources they need to accomplish the goals they set for themselves. Eliminating the symptoms of PTSD is no exception. With the NSA brainwave training, you will learn to enter into the powerful inner states of creativity and inventiveness and start the rebuilding of social skills; you will put an end to the trauma that was part of your past.

PTSD03 – Eliminate the Negative Effects of PTSD
It's important to understand that your mind is doing the best it can with the information it has at hand. During this session, you will train your brain to accept, use and benefit from new information. This new information will help you to become a software engineer for your own mind. Isn't it time you take back your personal power and write your own mental programs that bring back the joy, happiness and wonder to your life? This is all possible as you learn to use the most powerful computer on earth...your human brain. Today is the day you start to live again. One day at a time.

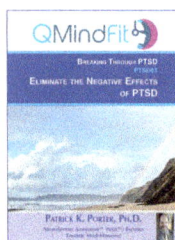

PTSD04 – Putting the Pieces Together After Trauma
This session was designed to integrate and heal the fracture that traumatic events cause. It is not uncommon for a person after such experiences to have feelings of abandonment and separation from who they thought themselves to be. The healing begins as you bring these different parts of yourself together. During this power session, you will begin to mentally rebuild the inner relationships that bring trust, honesty and self-confidence back into your life. True inner peace starts with you and expands out into your world. With this program you will experience the galvanizing effect of looking at your situation from a fresh perspective. You will discover that the past has no power over you. And you can create the balance you desire as early as today.

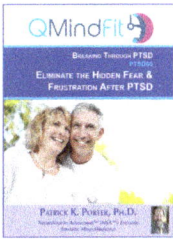

PTSD05 – Eliminate the Hidden Fear & Frustration After PTSD

Life is a series of choices, but when it feels as if every choice has a negative outcome, it becomes hard to make a change. This is why Dr. Porter created this program: to eliminate the uncertainty that can haunt you from past experiences. As you learn to plan, program and produce changes in your life, you will begin to trust the processes of life again. With the seeds of hope, you can grow the strength of a redwood to handle life's problems. You will discover what the great inventors of the past knew intuitively: if you have a problem in your life, your unconscious mind can solve it. Inventors like Tesla and Einstein would go to sleep with a problem and wake up with a solution. You can do the same!

PTSD06 – Developing Hope as a Habit; Moving Beyond PTSD

Habits are programs that were written either by design or default. During this Strategic Mind Messaging session, you will learn to design your destiny. When you set your goal on eliminating the effects of PTSD, your powerful mind can create healthy habits like hope and optimism. You will discover a flow state during this program that will allow you to remain relaxed even around the most difficult people and even under situations out of your control. You will discover the power of living a life of choice not of chance. It all starts with thoughts. You will set up a series of positive triggers that will keep you focused on personal success.

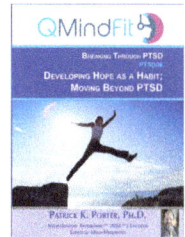

PTSD07 – Using Forgiveness as a Resource

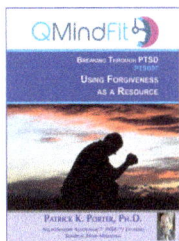

Healing trauma happens on many levels. You will experience the healing benefits of forgiveness so you can move with a sense of flow to the next phase of your life. No one can change the events of the past. But you can change the way your mind recalls them. With this simple yet profound session, you will learn key phrases that will help to change your internal dialogue so that you can once and for all release the past and begin to expect good things to happen in your life again.

PTSD08 – Creating the Relaxation Response

When Hubert Benson coined the term relaxation response, he thought the brain was hard-wired for fight or flight for coping with stress. We now know this isn't true, and that you can learn the relaxation response as a way to feel the stress and then move through it to release the pressure. This session is designed as an exercise where you will work with your mind and body, removing the built up kinetic energy and creating a reservoir of relaxation that will inoculate you against everyday stress. Once you learn this technique, you will be empowered to enjoy life in ways you thought unavailable to you since the trauma happened.

PTSD09 – Using the Theater of Your Mind to Reframe Your Past

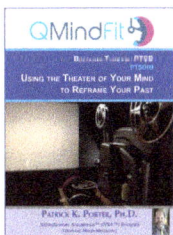

Reframing is a term used to describe looking at a situation in a new context. When trauma happens, it can affect your relationships, interaction with your family, and your experiences with friends. It can cause you to start destructive habits like drugs or alcohol. It's been said that all unhappiness stems from unfavorable comparisons. This is especially true for the PTSD sufferer. Dr. Porter will use this process to help you separate the stimulus from the response so you are not subject to old patterns or beliefs and are free to create a new future based on new experiences. You will appreciate the truth of knowing that you get what you rehearse in life, not necessarily what you intend. With the theater of the mind, you will be given a safe place to experiment with new behaviors. With this new experience, you can use the behaviors that work and eliminate those that don't.

Smoking Cessation Series
Patrick K. Porter, Ph.D.

Kicking your smoking habit doesn't get any easier or more fun than this! When you use Dr. Patrick Porter's proven strategies, you'll find that making this life-saving change comes about simply and effortlessly. With the new science of creative visualization and relaxation (CVR), you will extinguish the stress and frustration associated with quitting smoking, and you'll conquer your cravings like the tens of thousands of others who have used his processes.

You will learn to stay calm so you can easily and comfortably vanquish the old urge for cigarettes. Breaking the chains that have bound you to cigarettes has never been easier—now that you have made the choice to live your life tobacco-free and to start living the life of your dreams!

SS01 – Making the Decision To Be A Non-Smoker
Have you always wanted to quit smoking, but never had the confidence to take that plunge? With this CVR session, you'll learn about the cleansing power of you own mind, and use it to take a "mental shower" that will wipe away all thoughts of tobacco. With this process, you'll gladly make the decision to be tobacco-free for life!

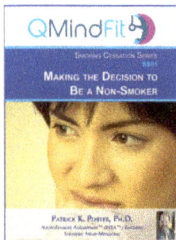

SS02 – Making Peace With Your Mind
In this powerful creative session, Dr. Patrick Porter will show you that, while you once had a positive intention for having tobacco in your life, you no longer need it to live the life you desire. The smoker of the past will make peace with the clean air breather of the future in order to create a new, vibrant you! This mind-blowing technique will allow you to learn from your past, master your present, and accomplish all your future goals.

SS03 – Plan Your Life As A Non-Smoker
Every goal needs a plan, and in this process, Dr. Patrick Porter will guide you in visualizing and working a plan for your tobacco-free life. This motivational session will allow you to remember to forget cigarettes forever. You'll awake convinced being a nonsmoker is as easy as taking a breath of fresh air!

SS04 – Freedom From Tobacco At Work
You will get a handle on negative emotions such as anger, stress, and frustration. At the same time, you'll release any triggers that could potentially cause you to return to the old unwanted behavior. This process is specifically designed to help you learn new ways to handle daily breaks, drive time, and times when your co-workers might be smoking around you. Imagine the power of saying with a smile, "No, thanks, I am a non-smoker!"

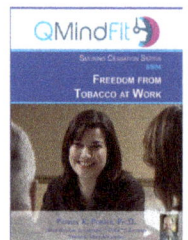

SS05 – Craving-Free/Tobacco-Free
Dr. Patrick Porter will help you learn effective new ways for releasing the chains that have bound you to the habit of smoking. When you think like a "non-smoker" you will find it easy to remain free from tobacco even while driving, when walking out of smoke-free buildings, or after dinner. Cravings will become a thing of the past as you employ the world's greatest computer...your human mind!

SS06 – Rid Your Mind of Stress & Frustration
Imagine learning exciting new ways to rid yourself of the two main foes that have prevented you in the past from being tobacco-free forever. Dr. Patrick Porter has trained thousands to use these success strategies to eliminate stress and frustration, and now he is going to help you. When you use the power of your mind, it becomes easy to handle even the most difficult situations.

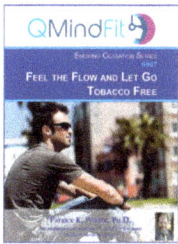

SS07 – Feel the Flow and Let Go - Tobacco-Free

You will tap into that innate intelligence that is greater than your conscious mind and release any anger that in the past may have driven you back to the smoking habit. With this process, you will learn visualization techniques of self-discipline and self-confidence that will train you to remain 100% tobacco-free for the rest of your life.

SS08 – Count Down to Being Tobacco-Free

During this creative visualization process, Dr. Patrick Porter will train you in techniques that will have you creating new triggers for health. As you develop self-discipline and self-confidence you will find the old negative triggers disappearing while a new life filled with health and abundance becomes yours.

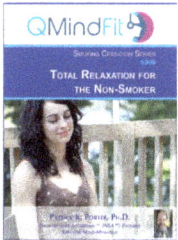

SS09 – Total Relaxation For The Non-Smoker

Relaxation is the key to transforming your new thoughts into action. Dr. Patrick Porter will help you gain the tools you need to be a non-smoker in day-to-day life. Best of all you will use the power of relaxation to transform stress into positive energy that will help you accomplish your goals. It is easy when you use your mind to simply relax away your cravings!

SS10 – Thinking Like A Non-Smoker

"Non-Smokers" think differently and you will learn how they avoid the usual quitting traps. With this breakthrough insight you will find it easy to remove the unwanted thoughts of tobacco forever. All permanent change starts in the mind and as you allow your mind to return to its natural way of thinking it will be as natural as your heart beat to remain tobacco-free.

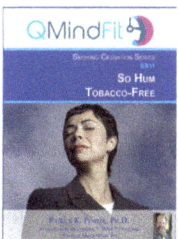

SS11 – So Hum Tobacco-Free

Dr. Patrick Porter will train you to change your thoughts as easily as changing the channel on your television. With this breathing technique and creative visualization you will discover the power of selective thinking so you can remove your cravings and accentuate the positive of living tobacco-free. You will notice that energy flows where attention goes. As you place your attention on health and positive living, the unseen forces of your mind will support you in making this change permanent.

SS12 – Problem Solving As A Non-Smoker

Stress is one of the main reasons people smoke. In this creative visualization process, Dr. Patrick Porter trains you to creatively handle stress and create solutions in your life—solutions that will make it easy to stay tobacco-free. Once you learn these powerful techniques, you will use them in other areas of your life to become a conscious creator so you can accomplish each and every one of your goals.

SS13 – Healthy Mind For A Tobacco-Free Lifestyle

Dr. Patrick Porter will teach you a quick three-step process for thinking and acting healthfully. When you create your perfect place of relaxation, de-stressing and conquering deadly habits like smoking is easy. After that, you can focus the power of possibility thinking on other goals you have for your life!

Children's Opportunity for Brilliance
Autism Series

JoQueta Hayes-Handy MS, CCC-SLP, President, Children's Opportunity for Brilliance, a Nonprofit Organization, has teamed up with Patrick K. Porter, Ph.D. developer of Self-Mastery Technology (SMT), to help create a breakthrough in learning for autistic children.

The Children's Opportunity for Brilliance—Autism Series is designed for autistic children. The series combines the COB learning system with the brain science of frequency following response using sound frequencies, spoken word and light frequencies to balance the brain (Q MindFit Neuro-Trainer™ required for lights).

This breakthrough technology can help to transform a dominant right brain learner into a whole brain thinker. Using the mind tools of rhythm, movement and visualization, each session engages the student to exercise the brain and balance the nervous system. The results are a relaxed and more focused mental environment optimized for learning. While the brainwave technology is helping balance your child's brain to remain in the optimum learning state, they will also be forming a habit of interpreting information in a useful way.

While each session builds upon the other, your child will practice correctly putting together sound sequences. When used with the Q MindFit Neuro-Trainer, your child's visual processing will also be exercised, leading to quick and easy understanding of what is seen and improving the ability to picture things in the mind. This is key to remembering what is seen and then verbalizing it.

It is a proven fact that whether an activity is done mentally or physically, the same neuron's fire. Through these visualization exercises, the autistic child learns to coordinate movement with what is seen in the mind's eye and then experienced as body movement. This is called linking. The series is designed to build new neural pathways so the new information gets linked to your child's prior knowledge for faster learning and better retention. Additionally, poor sleep patterns will become a thing of the past as your child's brain is exercised with the Q MindFit technology.

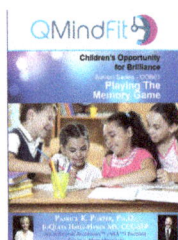

COB01 – Playing the Memory Game

Dr. Patrick K. Porter (PHD) has designed this first mind game to challenge the learner to adopt memory strategies that have a proven effect in improving short-term and long-term memory. With these lighthearted stories, your child will discover creative ways to recall auditory information for overall memory improvement.

COB02 – Tuning Your Brain, Hearing Your World…
Auditory Processing

Thanks to JoQueta's breakthroughs, developed over years of one-on-one work with autistic kids, your child will start engaging a whole-brain state for identifying sounds and symbols. With a focus on sound discrimination, this session provides the mind-time needed to build words from individual sounds. By exercising this skill at the other-than-conscious level of the mind, your child will be building the ability to sustain auditory attention, along with the ability to better discriminate the sounds they hear, a skill that will continue to improve. This in turn helps to eliminate the frustration of being unable to express needs or communicate in general.

COB03 – Adjusting Your Mind Lens, Seeing Your World

During this brain game, your child will experience accelerated visual processing exercises. Through the use of these COB exercises, letter and number recognition will improve. With the formation of numbers and letters, you will see your child's fine motor skills improving. As your child's confidence grows, a sense of accomplishment and pride will lead to setting goals and achieving them. Some of the results will be in the ability to see words and numbers as meaningful units and to understand the difference between b's and d's or p's and q's.

COB04 – Making the Connection, Processing Your World

Processing speed affects how the brain organizes information. During this brain game, Dr. Porter will help your child focus on important things while ignoring what is less important. This will help your child discover how the brain is able to shift from one activity to another. Your child will discover there are many ways the brain receives information. And during this fun adventure we will use both auditory and visual input, the two most common ways students receive and process information.. The goal of this session is to improve overall processing speed. Students should start to see improvement in test taking skills along with improvements in the ability to block out distracting, interfering sounds, with a key focus on distinguishing one voice from another. The side benefit of each session is your child will better remember what was heard. You will be amazed at the improvement in working memory and interaction with peers. Parents regularly report that their child is more comfortable in social situations.

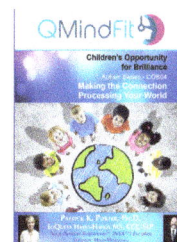

COB05 – Tuning Out Negative Thoughts and Trying New Things

Anxiety is highly prevalent among children with autism, along with obsessive and ritualistic behaviors. During this brain training, your child will learn how to eliminate obsessions and compulsions that are producing a negative response. If you find your child's mind is constantly whirring with thoughts, worries and concerns, this process can make all the difference. Autistic children commonly experience unwanted and intrusive thoughts that they can't seem to get out of their heads (obsessions), often compelling them to repeatedly perform ritualistic behaviors and routines (compulsions) to try and ease their anxiety. While playing this mind game, we work with your child to break this pattern by creating comfort in change.

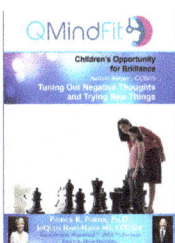

COB06 – Playing the Theater Game

The ability to shift gears from one thought to the next and plan out activities is key to executive function. In this session, Dr. Porter will help guide the listener by assigning goals, then working within the theater of the mind to practice achieving them. Whether the goal is reading, adding numbers or expressing ideas with the written word, playing the theater game will help build attention and focus in and out of the classroom.

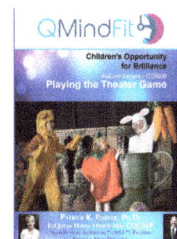

COB07 – Playing the Relationship Game

One of the main goals of the Children's Opportunity for Brilliance series is to accelerate brain activities that allow your child to set goals, organize, and complete tasks. These are skills required for any action or task that we do. During this process, your child will rehearse using executive functioning. This is the how of knowledge. It refers to the brain functions dedicated to how a child cleans his room or plays pirate. Shifting cognitive set refers to your child's ability to think about one activity and then shift thinking to another activity.

COB08 – Playing the Focus Game in Education

During this program, your child will learn impulse control. This is required to prevent distraction, and to keep your child focused on the appropriate task or step so that the goal can be reached. Inhibition is needed for sustained attention. It is also needed for delayed gratification. While listening to this brainwave entrainment session, your child will develop the capacity to wait until later before engaging in a preferred activity or before receiving a reward. Planning refers to the ability to order steps into a logical sequence so that a goal is reached. Whether that goal is reading comprehension, reading fluency, computation, written expression or sustaining attention, your child will mentally rehearse these steps until they become natural in everyday activities.

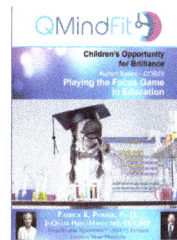

COB09 – Playing the Language Game Using Your Whole Brain

This session is designed for those children having difficulty linking thoughts and communicating ideas at a conversational level. Difficulty communicating emotions, expressive language delay, and not picking up on social cues—inference, sarcasm, facial expressions—are at the root of this issue. During this guided imagery session, Dr. Porter will help your child in expressing details and describing objects and events. Your child will learn to operate from a place of choice instead of fear. When children know where their bodies are in space and time, they can better go with the emotional flow. You will notice heightened self-esteem as negative associations around learning melt away. And best of all, homework time—usually a negative experience—will be transformed into productive time.

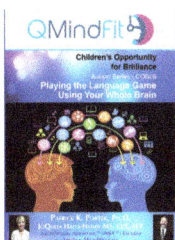

Enlightened Children Series
Patrick K. Porter, Ph.D.

Seven-year-old Marina Mulac and five-year-old Morgan Mulac, who have come to be known as the world's youngest marketers, were the inspiration behind this Enlightened Children's Series. When they met Dr. Patrick Porter, they had one question for him: Why had he created so many great visualizations for grown ups and nothing for kids?

Dr. Porter told the two little entrepreneurs that if they put on their thinking caps and helped him design a program for kids, together they could help children from around the globe to use their imaginative minds to become better people and help improve the world. Together, Marina, Morgan, and Dr. Patrick Porter put together this series that uses guided imagery, storytelling, and positive affirmations to help children see the world as a peaceful and harmonious place where everyone can win. If your goal is to develop a happy, healthy child of influence in our rapidly changing world, this series is a must-have for your child.

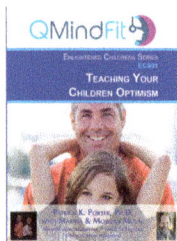

ESC01 – Building Optimism in Your Children
Every day your child is forming his or her view of the world based on life experiences. Now is the time to help your child build a positive outlook that will serve him or her for a lifetime. Optimists believe that people and events are inherently good and that most situations work out for the best. Dr. Porter will show your child how to see the good in every situation and how to be open to experiencing new things.

ESC02 – Developing Honesty as a Habit
With the influence of video games, movies, and television, it may sometimes be hard for children to identify true honesty. Dr. Porter will help your child realize that honesty is a way of communicating and acting truthfully in relation to the situations your child is in. This includes how he or she listens, speaks, and behaves around others.

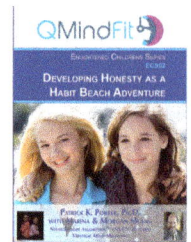

ESC03 – Flying the Kite of Kindness
With this guided imagery your child will go to an imaginary park to fly a kite. While the wind takes hold of the kite, the child learns why kindness is a virtue and how to let his or her innate kindness shine for all to see. By the time your child has finished flying the kite, he or she will understand that kindness reaps the reward of kindness in return.

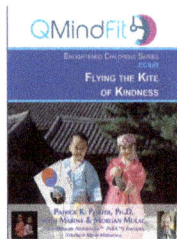

ECS04 – Playing the Change Game
Today's children live in a world that is changing daily. How well children learn to adapt to change will have a direct influence on his or her ability to cope with the stresses of our modern world. In this visualization your child will come to understand change as a natural part of life and will learn the skills to master it.

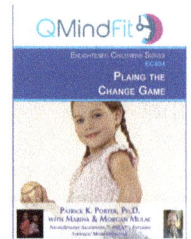

ECS05 – Nurturing a Love of Learning
With distractions such as video games and hundreds of television channels to choose from, it's no wonder children get easily bored in a learning environment. During this guided imagery session your child will plant the seeds of curiosity that will develop into an excitement about learning new things.

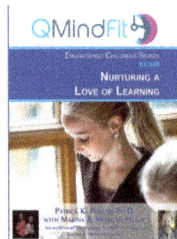

ECS06 – Making Exercise Fun
America has become a sedentary fast food nation. Consequently, the childhood obesity rate is soaring and along with it a plethora of weight-related health problems. It is the intention of this visualization to build a strong desire in your child to be physically active every day. When exercise becomes a way of life for your child, he or she will never have to endure the embarrassment and health risks associated with excess weight.

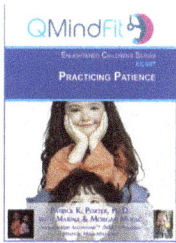

ECS07 Practicing Patience

Patience involves endurance during challenging situations; it means persevering in the face of delay and remaining calm while in the throes of provocation. Patience refers to the character trait of steadfastness. Wanting everything right now is a very real trait of the child in each of us. This session will help your child discover that life unfolds over time and that their needs are met when the time is right.

ESC08 – Visualize Peace in the World

The annual World Healing Day movement that started on December 31, 1986 at Noon Greenwich time has impacted thousands of lives for more than two decades. To further that directive, Dr. Porter has created this visualization where your child envisions the peace he or she wants to see in the world by developing that peace within.

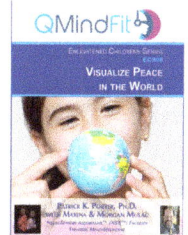

ESC09 – Respecting Yourself Respecting Others

During this visualization your child will gain a sense of self-worth and develop the ability to see that worth in others. Every child is special and is imbued with unique talents and attributes. Through this process children learn to enjoy sharing their special gifts with the world.

ESC10 – Being the Light of Leadership

Helping your child to become a leader instead of a follower is so important in today's rapidly advancing society. In this process Dr. Porter, with the help of Marina and Morgan, will help your child develop the ability to have a positive influence on others. This skill will help your child enlist the aid and support of others for accomplishing goals and will create an inner vision wherein he or she stays true to healthy and positive values.

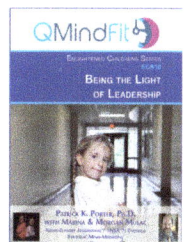

ESC11 – Bringing Compassion to the World

In this visualization Dr. Porter will help your child understand one of the greatest virtues — compassion. As your child comes to understand this profound human emotion, he or she will become motivated to take action and make a difference. Compassion is often the key component to altruism and is embodied by the golden rule: Do unto others as you would have done to you.

ESC12 – Being the Gift of Love

One of Dr. Porter's mentors, Dr. Jerry DeShazo, was inspired to share The Gift of Love with the world. This is a spiritual poem that can be read at http://www. theGiftofLove.com. Your child will learn this powerful visualization so that he or she can embody that gift in every word and deed.

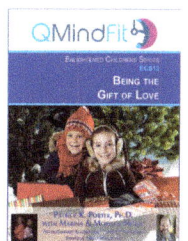

ESC13 – Building Healthy Relationships

This session focuses on the basic components of healthy relationships: expectations and communication. In this session your child will learn to identify with healthy relationships and will build that expectancy into developing healthy friendships. It is also designed to open communication between you and your child.

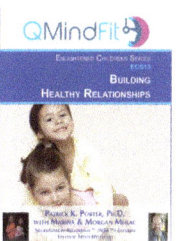

Marina & Morgan Mulac

In 2007, at the ages of 4 and 6, Marina Mulac and Morgan Mulac became the youngest marketers to ever grace the World Internet Main Event Stage in San Francisco, California when they were invited to report the results of their www.MommysBirthday.com fire sale, which grossed an unprecedented $8200.00 in one week for the two mini marketers. Quickly realizing the power of the Internet to touch lives, they are following in their parents footsteps and as a family they travel the U.S. speaking at marketing and motivational seminars while enjoying the home school lifestyle. Teaming up with Dr. Porter, their goal with the "Enlightened Children's Series" is to help children from around the globe to use their imaginative minds to become better people and help improve the world.

Optimizing Your Child's Inner Potential

This series was designed in partnership with Dr. Jared A. Leon, DC CCEP FICPA. Dr. Leon, with his specialty in neurology and physiology, and after using the Q MindFit Neuro-Trainer with patients and family members, saw a need for Self-Mastery Technology sessions for the pre-teen to young adult age group. He approached Dr. Patrick K. Porter, Ph.D. with his innovative concepts for promoting healthy childhood development and a collaboration was born.

This series is designed to help children understand, from the inside out, how powerful their minds truly are. It consists of nine sessions, each one focusing on a different life skill today's children will need to succeed and flourish in the fast-paced, rapidly evolving, 21st Century. This series bridges the gap between the Enlightened Children's Series for small children and the Accelerated Learning series for adults.

OYC01 – Mastering Homework with a Positive Mood

Throughout this brainwave entrainment session, children learn the value in correct breathing. They then learn the proper mindset for setting the mood and getting homework to the finish line. They will discover how easy it is to smile and think of something fun to do after homework is complete. In other words, they remember to start with an end in mind. With a powerful sense of accomplishment, they will try their best and stay focused on the task at hand. Asking for help is a key to success in school and life. Through the playing of this session, they will learn how to ask, how stay positive and they'll know they are loved and appreciated. During this session the other-than-conscious will help them understand that their parents are proud of them, which encourages them to keep up the great work.

OYC02 – Planning Happy Days at School

While children experience this brainwave entrainment session, they will also discover how to make learning fun. This session places special focus on being a great listener with all teachers. They learn to properly sort memories, stay positive while having great times with their friends, and create great memories for their future. Learning a life skill known as future-pacing, they will visualize being friendly to everyone they meet. A balanced life includes having fun, being physically active and playing at recess, eating a healthy lunch, and smiling often, especially at the end of the day, skills your child will develop through practice mentally as well as physically.

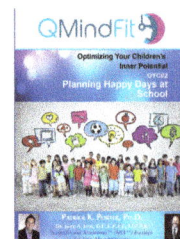

OYC03 – Mastering Confidence to Amplify Your Day

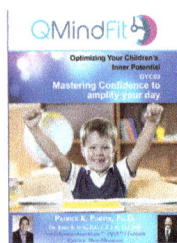

Dr. Jared Leon discovered that confidence starts with the inner knowledge that you are loved. During this session, your child will explore self-love and begin to own it. When they drift off into sleep, they will concentrate on the truth that they are special. They will build the belief that they are excellent at many things. As they develop that smart and witty attitude, people will enjoy their company. They will awaken the motivation to be a great starter and finisher of projects. As they develop this positive confidence, their friends will like being around them.

OYC04 – Having Fun and Laughing Often

It is said that laughter is the best medicine. During this brain training, children learn to have at least one belly laugh a day. While the mind plans this healthy activity, they will realize that laughter is an easy way to feel good. As they practice building the skill of smiling and laughing often, they will help others laugh as well (when appropriate). They will discover that laughter makes them feel great, that healthy laughter creates happiness and is one element to having fun daily. Mental practice at having fun makes them smile and be charismatic and allows their brains to work better.

OYC05 – Making Friends Easily

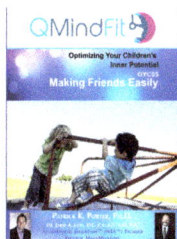

Those who have healthy friendships as children tend to be happier, more outgoing and more successful adults. During this session, children focus on the benefits of being kind and loving toward other children and how to recognize when other children want to be friends with them. They learn how a simple smile attracts others to them, and how to express a friendly confidence, knowing it is contagious to others. They rehearse making excellent eye contact, connecting with new friends easily, and bringing out the best in their friends. Learning how friends are always there for each other is a skill that forms children into balanced, contented adults.

OYC06 – Stimulating your Inner Creative Curiosity

Asking questions is the best way to learn. During this session, children learn to be curious about their surroundings while appreciating the beauty in all they see and experience. They come to recognize how curiosity helps nourish the creative genius within. They learn to aspire to self-awareness as they seek answers and truth. When children learn to spark their inner creative curiosity, they develop an inquisitive mind and an interest in learning and creating new things.

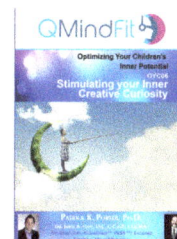

OYC07 – Your Parents Magically Know Best

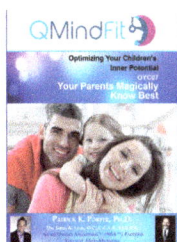

Children usually view parents as a vehicle for testing boundaries and learning limits. Unfortunately, in doing so, they often develop negative habits such as acting out and pushing buttons. During this session, children learn positive, healthy ways to interact with parents. They come to understand that parental decisions are based on love and appreciation and that parents always have their best interests at heart. They learn that growing up is easier and more fun when you listen to your parents and, most importantly, to have gratitude for the amazing parents they have. Life is easier for children who allow their parents to guide them through the childhood journey because parents have already made the silly mistakes they can learn from. Through parental love, children learn to become loving and caring adults.

OYC08 –Happy Mornings and Happy Bus Rides

Children who wake up with a positive expectancy for a wonderful day tend to develop a healthy, optimistic outlook. While children experience this harmonizing brainwave entrainment process, they will rehearse waking up happy, getting dressed with excitement for a great day, eating a healthy breakfast to enrich their brains and bodies, and completing all chores and morning rituals before going to school. They will learn to be respectful to all family members and to say a positive affirmation either with the family or by themselves. Every member of the family benefits when children awaken in a good mood, are ready and on time, and look at the bus ride to school as a chance to meet someone new or share quality time with good friends.

Diabetes Active Lifestyle Program
Patrick K. Porter, Ph.D.

Diabetes affects 26 million Americans, it is likely that you know someone who has diabetes, and perhaps you may be the one who has diabetes. Now Dr. Patrick Porter (PhD) has partnered with Owen Durkin a researcher and father of a child with diabetes to help others manage the stress of this lifestyle disease. It is said, "You don't have to like diabetes, you just have to get along with it", and that is just what you are going to do! Follow these 10 transformative sessions and make the management and navigation of your diabetes easier.

DAL01 – Activate Your Daily Plan for an Active Life-style

Your daily management plan is your key to the complication-free, active lifestyle you imagine yourself enjoying. PWD's spend an average of less than 6 hours a year in consultation with their diabetic caregivers, meaning that the responsibility of managing your condition lies primarily with you. Diabetes is a serious health challenge, but it is one that can be managed successfully. New advances in treatment and technology make it easier for PWD's (persons with diabetes) to enjoy healthy, complication-free lives.

DAL02 – Stimulate Your Daily Commitment

When combined with your own personal commitment to an effective daily management plan, these tools and technologies, which have become more affordable and accessible than ever, are your allies against both the long term, and short term effects of diabetes. There are a number of keys to preventing complications and preventing the onset of disruptive symptoms which can affect your quality of life both physically, and emotionally.

DAL03 – Being Proactive In Your Daily Diabetes Management

It is important to be proactive as opposed to being reactive, in terms of your daily management plan. You can do this by taking steps to understand the fundamentals of successful diabetes management. Frequent monitoring allows you to treat fluctuations in blood glucose in a timely manner, and to avoid unpleasant side effects. But it does much more than that. It also gives you tremendous insight into how effective your management strategy really is. By monitoring the effects of your dosages, your caregiver can help you calculate the amounts of medication you require. It also reveals patterns and trends in one's blood glucose levels.

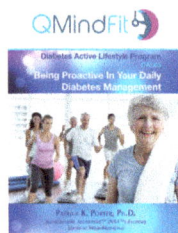

DAL04 – Personal Choice; Your Commitment to a Complication-Free Life

Every PWD is unique, with specific treatment requirements that are specifically calibrated to their own needs, by a qualified diabetes caregiver. Implementing the strategy comes down to personal choice and commitment to a complication-free life. A simple log book is a powerful tool in keeping track of blood glucose readings and corresponding timings, which a trained caregiver can interpret in order to help you refine your personal management plan. Logging other types of data will also help you to maintain healthy and safe blood glucose levels. By tracking the amount of carbohydrates in the foods you eat, as well as quantities, you can build your own simple, yet powerful database of information.

DAL05 – Consistency; Your Key Successful Diabetes Relief

The key to successful management is consistency. Maintaining consistency requires high levels of mental discipline. Feelings of despair, frustration, and mental fatigue associated with the struggles of maintaining optimal health can impair the ability and desire to be diligent with your management strategy. These lingering ideas can occasionally lead to lapses in judgment. You may sometimes find yourself deliberately choosing to "defy" your condition by deliberately neglecting your management strategy.

DAL06 – Doing Your Part to Keep Blood Sugar Level

You may choose to avoid testing your glucose or "skip" needles or boluses. You may begin to guess concerning required insulin dosages, or perhaps you will become comfortable with (or accustomed to) frequent swings from high to low blood glucose levels, which place an unnecessary strain on your body, your vital organs, and your general well being. This habit may eventually de-sensitize you and impair your ability to feel the onset of a hypoglycemic episode, which could prove to be dangerous. This kind of discipline can be fostered and fortified through choosing internal representations that support the end goal of good disease management practices, and provide a stable anchor when you are challenged by circumstances which may otherwise overwhelm you. You may choose to indulge frequently in less than nourishing foods, avoid carrying emergency glucose, or avoid wearing a medical alert product. You may even develop a drug, nicotine, or alcohol dependency to cope with the burden of life with diabetes.

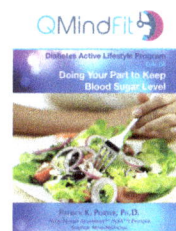

DAL07 – Eliminate Failure as an Option

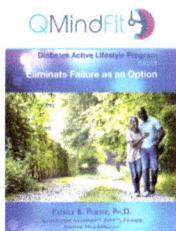

What I want to offer is an alternative to the endless strain of fighting what may at times feel like a losing battle, those self imposed incriminations for "failing" to take care of yourself, and the need to compensate by undertaking actions that increase your chances of a health crisis. If you are ready to entertain the notion that things can be much, much better, that you can reclaim your life and your sense of wellbeing, that you can be active and symptom-free for years to come, then allow me to re-introduce you to your most important piece in your management strategy: your mind.

Freedom from Irritable Bowel Syndrome
Patrick K. Porter, Ph.D.

When Dr. Patrick Porter (Ph.D.) was asked by his clients to help with Irritable Bowel Syndrome (IBS) back in the early 1980's he first thought that relaxation technique could help this problem. Then a client brought in a series of magazine articles showing that in the United Kingdom the first thing a medical doctor would do is refer them to a therapist for creative imagery and relaxation training.

This is when his quest to help his clients with this common problem with the intestines began. It is believed that in most cases IBS is more of a thinking problem than a physical problem where a person's intestines squeeze too hard or not hard enough and cause food to move too quickly or too slowly through the intestines. IBS usually begins around age 20 and is more common in women.

IBS01 – Mental Tips on Controlling Your IBS Symptoms

During this foundation session Dr. Porter teaches you to take the time to reduce your stresses and apprehensions. The key to relief is becoming familiar with the mind/body connection and to learn that you can eliminate the emotional triggers that put you out of control.

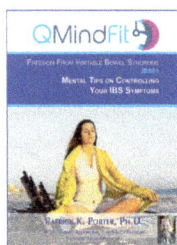

IBS02 – Being Physically & Mentally Balanced

This session helps the listener manage IBS symptoms by letting the users understand the benefits of allowing both mind and body to work together towards the goal of relief. Science has shown that the best way to handle IBS is to eat a healthy diet, avoid foods that seem to make you feel worse and find ways to handle your stress.

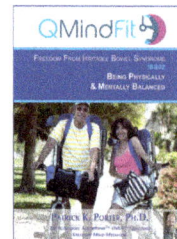

IBS03 – Stress Buster; Your Key to IBS Relief

With stress being a symptom that may cause the listener to get worse when they travel, attend social events or change their daily routine, Dr. Porter has created a simple technique that puts you instantly back in control. Our bodies are designed with the flight or fight response, but with the new science of Creative Visualization and Relaxation (CVR) you can learn the "Relaxation Response." This technique will work whether your symptoms get worse if you don't eat enough healthy foods or after you've eaten a big meal.

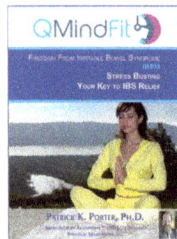

IBS04 – Using Your Mind to Regulate Your Body

You will learn to use the power of suggestion to enable to visualize the control and speed of peristaltic waves of the GI tract that will lead to a normal bowel movement. Whether you suffer from bloating and gas, the key is relaxation and to bring the body back into homeostasis. This can be done with proper diet and relaxation.

IBS05 – Staying True to Your Body for IBS Support

Food sensitivity can be a major cause of IBS and during this session Dr. Porter will guide you through mental exercises where you will plan to avoid the foods that cause the problem to worsen. You will also use visualization to creatively increase your fiber. Health science has discovered that fiber can be helpful because it improves how the intestines work. You will relax and plan to use the 2 types of fiber. Soluble fiber helps both diarrhea and constipation.

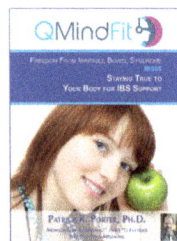

IBS06 – Tips on controlling IBS for a Healthy Life

In this self directed session you will learn a breakthrough technique that you can use to eliminate stress and stay focused on healthy living. Dr. Porter will reinforce the elimination of old stress that in the past triggered the old symptoms of IBS. You will build a time-line for change by building a support system including your family doctor or health care provider. This technique will help you if the symptoms get worse when you're under stress, such as when you travel, attend social events or change your daily routine. You will plan to eat a varied healthy diet and avoid foods high in fat and drink plenty of water.

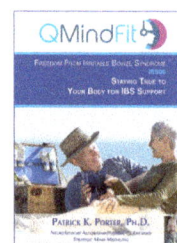

Gluten-Free Lifestyle
Patrick K. Porter, Ph.D.

Health experts from all sides of the nutrition spectrum, including weight loss specialists, bariatric physicians, and dietitians, are talking about the health benefits of a gluten-free diet, especially in light of the escalating number of people being diagnosed with celiac disease and gluten sensitivity. If you have gluten intolerance, a gluten-free diet can have a variety of health benefits, such as eliminating digestive problems, improving cholesterol levels, lowering blood sugar, and increasing energy.

Today, even people who don't have a gluten problem are opting for a gluten-free lifestyle because of the health benefits. For starters, eating gluten-free naturally eliminates the unhealthiest foods. For example, fried foods would be off limits, because of the breading, and desserts high in sugar and fat would be removed from your diet completely. On a gluten-free diet, you would likely eat more fruits and vegetables, because these are readily available food sources that are naturally gluten-free.

A gluten-free diet can help reduce your risk of heart disease, certain cancers, and other health-related conditions, like diabetes. A gluten-free diet can also help ward off viruses and germs, because many of the replacement foods you eat will be full of antioxidants, and essential vitamins and minerals. Needless to say, a gluten-free diet is a worthwhile endeavor, and this Q MindFit series will help make your transition to gluten-free easy and fun!

GFL01 – Stimulate Your Metabolism – Go Gluten-Free
During this Q MindFit session, you will super-charge your motivation to go gluten-free. It's never easy making a life change if stress is an overriding factor. Dr. Patrick Porter (PhD) will help you learn the relaxation response and quickly integrate this valuable change in your life. You will experience better results from exercise. Your cholesterol levels can return to normal. Seeking out healthy alternatives will have your energy improving and your waistline rapidly returning to normal.

GFL02 – Unlock Your Body's Health – Live Gluten-Free
Tapping into the innate healing potential of the body has never been easier. Dr. Porter will help you stay gluten-free and eliminate bloating and excessive gas. You will train your brain through neurosensory algorithms to avoid negative carbohydrates that have the reputation of being the meanest gas producing foods. Being gluten-free almost always has an added benefit of weight loss. You will tap into your own resource generator and focus on a gluten-free diet low in refined carbohydrates, so you can lose unwanted pounds while getting healthier.

GFL03 – Visualize Your Gluten-Free Lifestyle
Dr. Porter will help you create a timeline for becoming gluten-free, while helping you avoid the negative gluten-free foods that use cornstarch and other harmful fillers. Saying no to wheat and wheat products is only the first step as you boost your immune system and learn to control exorphins, which stimulate appetite. Throughout this process you will experience the natural benefits of the Q MindFit, with a more focused mind, better memory and improved concentration. You will begin noticing a calming effect on your nervous system, which will help eliminate nighttime cravings.

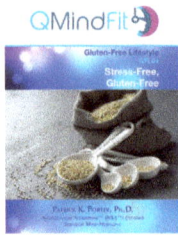

GFL04 – Stress-Free, Gluten-Free

Going gluten-free means your digestion is better; it also means that you are eliminating a powerful appetite stimulant. Dr. Porter will teach you a bulletproof method for saying no to wheat in three easy steps. The natural benefit will be the elimination of your wheat belly as your waistline returns to normal. You can expect improved heart health as insulin levels balance out, giving your pancreas a break. You will learn the quick facts that will keep you gluten-free for life. As the discomfort in your colon is relieved, you will start to enjoy life again.

GFL05 – Shopping Gluten-Free

At times it might seem you are working against yourself, with a part of you wanting to eat the gluten foods that caused the problems in the first place. Dr. Porter will help you eliminate the confusion that comes with making a positive lifestyle change. You will visualize eating more fresh fruits and vegetables to overcome the old carb cravings. As you learn to relax and change your diet, you will focus on the positive benefits like alkalizing your body, which equals fat burning, healthier bones and freedom from joint pain.

GFL06 – Eating Out Gluten-Free

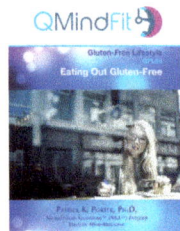

Being gluten-free separates you from the masses, so you need assertiveness skills to ask for what you want. Dr. Porter will share with you a technique to create your unlimited reality where you can look over any menu and pick out the gluten-free foods. Your self-esteem will be soaring as you realize that you are worth the time, energy and effort of staying gluten-free.

GFL07 – Gluten-Free Travel (Theater of the Mind)

Being gluten-free improves your balance and cognitive skills, but that doesn't stop life from presenting challenges to your new lifestyle. During this Q MindFit session, you will enter the theater of your mind and plan to succeed in any environment, instead of counting on failure. As you notice your higher brain functions improving, you will plan ahead with gluten-free foods on the top of your priority list. Your learning and memory improves as inflammation and pain go down. The Q MindFit will balance your mood and eliminate any withdrawal symptoms.

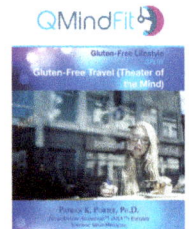

Heart Healthy Lifestyle
Patrick K. Porter, Ph.D.
Inspired by the principles of Dr. Michael Irving's

Twelve Wisdoms to a Healthy Heart

Adversities and life challenges can be viewed as burdens or as gifts. A heart attack or diagnosis of heart disease is a dramatic wakeup call. Dr. Porter and Dr. Irving want you to see your diagnosis as the gift that it is—the opportunity to create a heart-healthy lifestyle and a brand new you!

Twelve Wisdoms to a Healthy Heart is for individuals who wish to develop a heart-healthy lifestyle and prevent or reverse heart disease. This audio series introduces you to the guided visualization process for changing lifestyle habits, reducing stress, and creating a heart healthy lifestyle. You will begin by internalizing Dr. Irving's "Twelve Wisdoms to a Healthy Heart" which include: 1) Taking Charge, 2) Family and Friends 3) A Health Care Team, 4) Medicines and Supplements 5) Visualization, 6) Heart Healthy Food, 7) Exercise for Life, 8) Stress Reduction, 9) Listening to Your Heart, 10) Harmony and Balance, 11) Meditation and Relaxation , 12) A Spiritual Connection

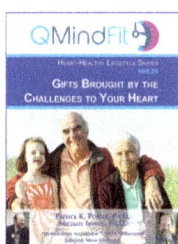

HHL01 – Gifts Found in Accepting the Challenges to Your Heart

A heart crisis can be frightening; but it can also make you feel grateful to be alive and can increase your appreciation of life. This first guided visualization helps you define important resolutions and then motivates you to take action. These early changes will have you well on your way to living a vibrant life of energy and vitality.

HHL02 – Take Charge with a Strong Heart

Taking charge is one of the most important components of heart health and recovery. Now you can take ownership of your own health and be the central director of your success, confident in your knowledge of heart health, and ready to make the decisions that fulfill your goals. Being in charge will make you feel strong at heart.

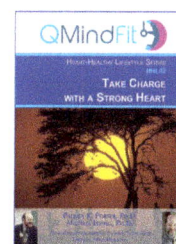

HHL03 – Opening the Heart to Family and Friends

The heart represents receiving and giving, loving and caring. Now you can move away from the isolation and disconnection that leads to stress and the toxic repercussion that is heart disease. After a cardiac crisis, it is not uncommon for loved ones to gather information and resources to help you. By accepting these gestures of genuine love and concern, you will be well on your way to healing. With this visualization, you will come to see family and friends as positive beacons of encouragement.

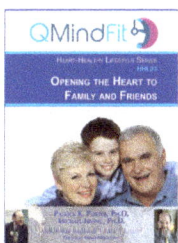

HHL04 – Gathering a Health Care Team for Your Heart

Now that you have taken charge, it's time to eliminate any blocks you have that inhibit you from communicating with your heart health experts. You will increasingly feel empowered to ask questions and gather all the information you need for an optimal recovery. Through this visualization you will learn to take full advantage of the wisdom your health care team offers.

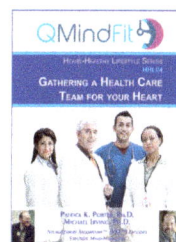

HHL05 – Medicines and Supplements for Heart Health and Recovery

Learning all you can about medicines, supplements, herbs, and remedies can help you prevent, manage, and reverse heart disease. Through this visualization, you will direct the power of your mind and body to work with your medicines and supplements for optimum effectiveness. You will also create an inner resolve and lock in a commitment to your heart-health regimen.

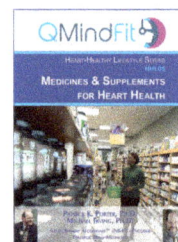

HHL06 – The Power of Visualization for Heart Health

Visualization brings the mind, body, and heart together. What a powerful tool for promoting wellbeing and change. This session creates and enhances positive feelings and helps you make the mind/body connection for healing. You will be directed to spontaneously visualize your heart-healthy lifestyle throughout your day, making positive life choices easy and natural.

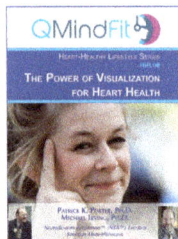

HHL07 – Heart Healthy Food for Life

A healthy heart needs fresh and vibrant foods. This session reinforces what your body already knows—fresh vegetables and whole foods make your heart and arteries healthy and vital. You will visualize your food as healing medicine while you plan, shop for, and cook your heart-healthy meals.

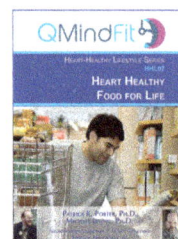

HHL08 – Strengthen the Heart with Exercise for Life

Exercise is a primary cornerstone of heart rehabilitation. Regular exercise helps clear the body of stress, builds muscle, strengthens the heart, cleans the arteries, promotes weight loss, and creates energy and vitality throughout the day. Through this visualization process, you will gain positive images of your physical fitness and you will be motivated to stay consistent with your exercise program.

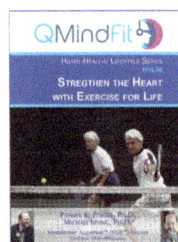

HHL09 – Stress Reduction to Calm the Heart

Stress subjects the body to persistent and elevated levels of adrenaline and cortisol, causing damage to the arteries and heart. With this creative visualization, you will listen to your inner voice to uncover what is at the root of your stress. This session will not bring you peace from the outside; rather, it will open you up to the tranquility already present within you.

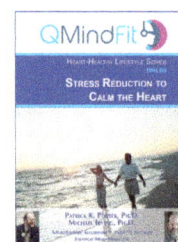

HHL10 – Listening to Your Heart

A gift of your cardiac crisis is that it poignantly points out the fragility of your life. When you are physically ill in your heart, you are also unwell in your essence. If you are feeling a heavy heart, simply listen to this process and learn to lighten it. Your heart will guide you toward your passions in life--all you have to do is listen.

HHL11 – Harmony and Balance for a Quiet Heart

Modern life is filled with demands and activities that throw us off balance and overwhelm us. Setting priorities is essential to managing the stresses of life. This process will help you find ways to ground yourself, have variety in your life, find time for pleasure and rest, manage your work life, and approach life activities with mindfulness so that you are living in the present moment.

HHL12 – Meditation and Relaxation for a Peaceful Heart

The heart requires periods of calm. With this visualization you will learn to achieve the relaxation response, a powerful key to releasing the natural healing forces of the brain and body. Through special meditations on your heart health, you will gain an inner strength and resolve. You will know there is a purpose for your life and that your life is abundant now and in the future.

HHL13 – Spiritual Connections from the Heart

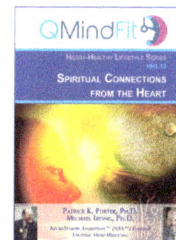

Heart, spirit, and soul are closely connected. The life-death confrontation of a cardiac incident increases your contemplation of meaning, purpose, and a higher power. It is no accident that you are still here. Through this visualization, you will be inspired by knowing that your cardiac crisis and has led you to the help you need so you can awaken to a better and more fulfilling life.

While watching a nail-biting Stanley Cup hockey game, Dr. Irving experienced a life threatening heart attack. The reality of his mortality quickly brought into perspective his busy lifestyle and unhealthy habits. So profound were the positive changes he made in his life, it led his rehab supervisor to say that in twenty-five years at one of North America's largest cardiac clinics she had never before seen such dramatic improvement across such a broad range of measures. In reflecting on what led to his impressive recovery, Dr. Irving realized that he had employed the "Twelve Wisdoms to a Healthy Heart" that you will discover here. By following Dr. Irving's lead, you too can be inspired to reverse heart disease and enjoy a life that you love.

The "Reaching Out Monument" was originally designed by Dr. Irving for the Northwest corner of College and University.

There have been many impressive endorsements for the architectural, aesthetic, cityscape, healing, educational and social appropriateness of this location.

Sarah Hood -- National Post

http://www.irvingstudios.com

Healthy Sleep Habits

More and more, stress and the inability to unwind and relax keeps people from getting the kind of restful sleep needed to awaken refreshed and rejuvenated. Many people don't even realize that stress and poor sleep habits is the root cause of their daytime drowsiness, irritability, lack of concentration, and poor memory. The body requires deep, restorative sleep to recharge and rebuild, and great sleep is a key ingredient to a great quality of life. In this audio series, Dr. Patrick Porter (PhD) will help you discover how, by using Q MindFit, you experience deep relaxation, which contributes to maintaining healthy sleep patterns and a fantastic quality of life.

IS01 – Sleep Deep and Awaken Recharged

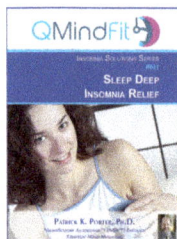

Did you know that you already possess the most powerful pharmacy on earth? It's the human mind. Through the power of thought, your brain easily produces the neurotransmitters that lead to the beneficial, quality sleep you need. In this session, by using creative visualization, Dr. Porter will guide you through the thought processes that will deliver the deepest states of relaxation and promote healthy, high quality sleep.

IS02 – Planning a Restful Night's Sleep

In this process, Dr. Porter will teach you to look forward to sleep. You will train your mind to think differently by easing the effects of any nervous tension at the approach of sundown, throughout the evening hours, and at bedtime. You will re-associate with the dreamy, drowsy state of sleepiness you've experienced in the past so that you can relax, unwind, and slip into deep, restorative sleep. And the Q MindFit visualization will help reverse the effects of any stressful events and eliminate negativity from your sleep cycle.

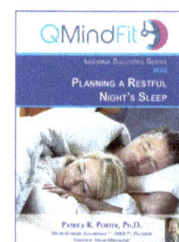

IS03 – Making Peace with Your Body for Deep Restful Sleep

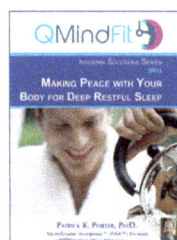

People who have poor sleep habits tend to be the same people who try to control situations, people, and events that are beyond their control. With this Q MindFit session, Dr. Porter will help you put your life into perspective so you can rediscover your natural sleeping patterns. You will release the unconscious need to react with fear, both consciously and unconsciously, about any situation that is not within your control. At the same time, through the relaxation response, you will be guided to a state of relaxation which is helpful in making natural physical changes such as slowing your heartbeat and regulating your breathing. You will experience the positive benefits of relaxation and it's assistance in attaining a good night's sleep.

IS04 – Sleep Deep and Let Go of Unwanted Fears Forever

During deep relaxation and sleep, physical changes occur that are a natural part of the process of falling into slumber. Feelings such as floating, being in a trance, or of a slowed heartbeat are common. These are natural parts of the sleep cycle. You will learn to allow these changes to guide you into deep sleep. Dr. Porter will teach a simple visualization and relaxation technique to help promote healthy sleep patterns and achieve a restful night's sleep.

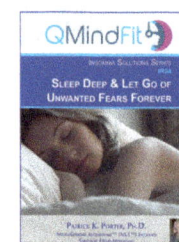

IS05 – Going with the Flow Day and Night

In this session, Dr. Porter will help you to counteract the stress that causes fears and frustrations that may be keeping you from a good night's rest. You will learn techniques that promote relaxation so you can rid yourself of anxious thoughts and worries. At the same time, new behaviors will disrupt past habits that may be causing you to physically react to stressful situations. Since you will no longer be mentally escalating negative thoughts and emotions during the day, you will be free to sleep comfortably all night long.

Natural Lyme Relief Breakthrough

Lyme disease, sometimes referred to as Lyme infection, is a bacterial illness, transmitted to humans by the bite of deer ticks carrying a bacterium known as Borrelia burgdorferi. Lyme is a systemic issue that can ruin lives. While the medical community seeks fast, effective treatment for the symptoms, Dr. Patrick Porter (PhD) designed "Natural Lyme Relief Breakthrough" with Charmaine Bassett (PSC, SC, NMD, DM), Chief of Nemenhah Seminaries Services.

Ms. Bassett has been working for over 35 years in the health/nutrition field alongside her parents, who own and operate two of the largest health food stores in Ohio. This allowed her to study with some of the industry's leaders and led her to the discovery of her own healing breakthroughs.

Charmaine has been using brain-wave entrainment since the late 1980's and worked directly with Dr. Porter in the creation of this series. Because there is always a lot of pain involved in Lyme disease, she recognized that by teaching sufferers to use the most powerful pharmacy on earth, their human brains, relief of these symptoms can be found.

The series is designed to guide the user through a series of mental exercises to balance brain waves and approach natural healing with a positive attitude, trusting that the power that made the body can heal the body.

LR01 – Deep Relaxation for Lyme Relief

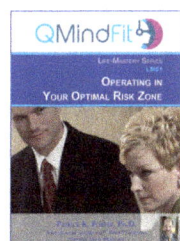

Although most people don't realize it, one of the most debilitating diseases of the modern world can often be found crawling around in the hedges, shrubs and tall grasses of the typical American backyard. Carried by several common species of tick, Lyme Disease - which leaves many victims struggling with long-term chronic illness, Post-Lyme Disease (PLD) - is one of the fastest-growing infectious-disease epidemics both here and abroad, according to recent research. With this session, you will train your brain to focus on the natural healing processes of the body while eliminating the trauma of the past experience. It has long been known that when your body is in the brain wave states of Alpha and Theta, the innate power to heal is more active in the body. You will learn the process of reframing past events and looking forward to a life full of energy as you release the past imprint of disease and accept the blueprint for health.

LR02 – Lyme Headache Relief

Even if you have bounced from physician to naturopath to herbalist to acupuncturist, or other non-traditional healers, there is still hope. During this session you will learn the relaxation techniques that will help you eliminate headache pain by turning on the most powerful pharmacy on earth, your human brain. Even if you have spent tens of thousands of dollars on treatments with little or no result, once you tap the innate intelligence of your body, there are no limits to what you can do.

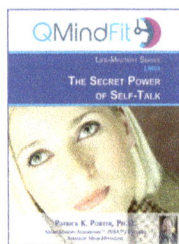

LR03 – Lyme Joint Pain Relief

While this bacteria-triggered illness leaves many of its victims struggling for years with fatigue, headaches, mental confusion, memory impairment, shortness of breath, sensitivity to bright light, abdominal pain, chronic muscle and joint pain--and several other nasty complaints, there is light at the end of the tunnel. As you learn to master the relaxation response, you will discover new ways to train your brain to master pain and live an active life without the discomfort of Lyme Disease.

LR04 – Supercharge Your Immune System

Through deep relaxation and brain wave entrainment, your symptoms of Post Lyme Disease can be eliminated and your immune system can be super-charged. During this session Dr. Porter will teach the techniques that cancer survivors use to boost their immune system.

LR05 – Rebuilding Your Natural Sleep Response

Many physicians feel that diagnostic tests for Lyme are unreliable; and all of this confusion leaves the Lyme sufferer with stress, worry and sleepless nights. Since the early 80s, Dr. Porter has been helping people to return to a natural deep sleep with the help of visualization and brainwave entrainment. During this session you will train the brain to return to its natural sleep cycle, allowing you to awaken rested, relaxed, revitalized and renewed.

LR06 – Relax and Listen To Your Heart

All too often, suffering patients have been left in the middle, essentially ignored by doctors who contend that their long-term symptoms aren't the result of Chronic Lyme, but of "fibromyalgia," "depression," or "irritable bowel syndrome." During this session, you can tune into innate intelligence and allow the power that made the body heal the body. Regardless of the diagnosis, the key is a heart healthy diet, positive thinking and deep relaxation to recharge the body.

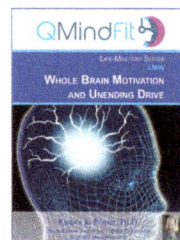

LR07 – Mind/Body Lyme Relief

Already struggling with the debilitating symptoms of their tick-borne disease, Post-Lyme sufferers are patronized with insulting regularity by professionals who don't understand the biochemistry involved in chronic, neurotoxin-mediated illnesses, of which PLD is only one. During this session you will learn to ask for what you need and build your support team so that you stay on the path to recovery.

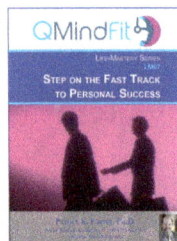

Mind-Over-Menopause
Patrick K. Porter, Ph.D.

For many women mid-life can be a time of uncertainty and loss. For some the loss of fertility and the perceived loss of youth can cause depression and anxiety. At the same time, the body's response to the decrease in hormones can create any number of symptoms—hot flashes, night sweats, weight gain, itchy skin, mood swings, lost libido, headaches, and irregular cycles are just of few of the menopausal challenges women face. In the midst of all these changes, relationships can suffer as loved ones start to ask, "What happened to the caring, loving woman we once knew?" Now you can reclaim that woman, along with all the strength, confidence, and wisdom you gained in the first half of your life. This series takes you way beyond mind over matter—it's mind over menopause!

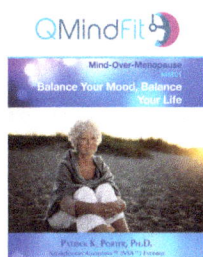

MM01 – Balance Your Mood, Balance Your Life

With this session you will use creative visualization and relaxation to help balance your mood, harness positive mental energy, and use your innate creative power to produce much-needed balance in your life during this time of change and uncertainty. You will stop focusing on what you've lost, and discover all that you've gained!

MM02 – Creating Harmony With the Cycles of Life

Using your mind, you will activate the powerful calming effects produced by your own brain chemistry. When you relax and let your mind experience a cascade of positive thoughts and images, you will find that the emotional ups and downs of menopause become a distant memory.

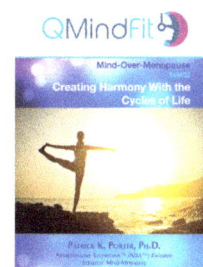

MM03 – Mental Skills to Help You Master Menopause

With this creative visualization and relaxation process, you will be given time to plan your life from a new perspective. You will learn to view menopause as a rite of passage—one that gives you confidence and inner worth.

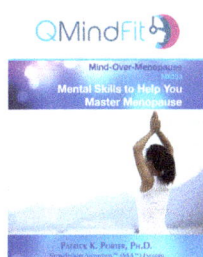

MM04 – Relax and Control Night Sweats and Hot Flashes

Now you can greatly reduce or eliminate the hot flashes and night sweats typically associated with menopause. Relaxation therapy is a natural remedy for hot flashes and many women have found lasting relief with this method. Now, with the added dimension of creative visualization, you will discover that you can master the cooling effects of your mind, and you will feel your body naturally cooling off as well!

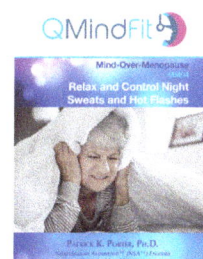

MM05 – Eliminate "Brain Fog" and Sharpen Your Memory

Has menopause got you in a fog? Do you sometimes wonder where your memory went? During menopause many women describe this lack of focus and concentration as "brain fog." When the fog sets in, sometimes even the easiest tasks can seem confusing or overwhelming.

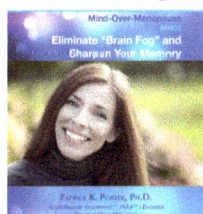

MM06 – Coping With Emotional Changes During Menopause

Get ready to see yourself as the woman you've chosen to be! In this session, you will be building healthy coping mechanisms for conquering mood swings, overcoming anxiety, and regaining your libido. Thanks to a little-known side benefit to deep relaxation, you will also notice improved concentration, soaring energy levels, and freedom from the irritability of the past.

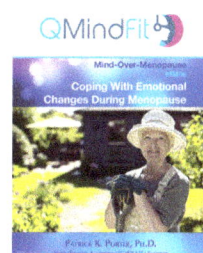

MM07 – Get Connected in Times of Uncertainty

Many menopausal women describe feeling disconnected from their bodies, as if they are suddenly uncomfortable within their own skins. Using your innate creativity, you will learn new tools to rid your mind of these confusing, and often unpleasant, thoughts and feelings. You will discover a new sense of connectedness and purpose, and your "woman's intuition" will be back in full swing!

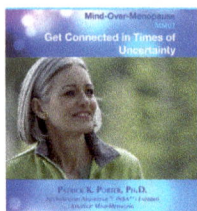

MM08 – Eliminate Fatigue and Boost Your Energy

Tap into the flow that is your personal power and feel your fatigue and low energy levels melt away. While relaxing with this process you will learn to own your own personal space and will develop an emotional drive to make your wellbeing a top priority.

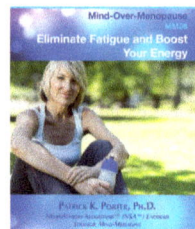

MM09 – Mastering the Physical Changes of Menopause

When you tap into the power of possibility thinking and engage the internal pharmacy within your brain. You can eliminate gastrointestinal distress, nausea and those dreadful headaches. During this session, you will put a plan into action for controlling weight gain, bloating, or that tingling, itchy skin so many women experience.

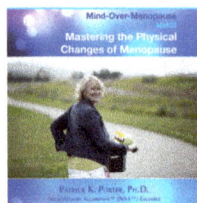

MM10 – Tips for Quick Menopausal Relief

Sometimes you need relief right now! This session is your answer. You can just sit back, relax and let these tips for reducing stress, clearing your head, and regrouping take you away. Within the session you will create a new, healthier lifestyle that includes cutting back on caffeine, alcohol, and spicy foods the easy way.

MM11 – Making Peace With Your Body

This session is like Tai Chi for the mind. Discover new ways to handle those unusual menopausal symptoms such as that annoying buzzing in your head, electric shock sensations, dry mouth, dry eyes, dizziness, or lightheadedness. When you learn to practice mental Tai Chi, the transition through mid-life and menopause can be far easier than you think!

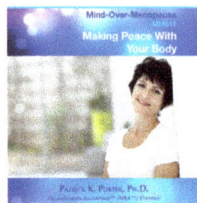

MM12 – Pain Control and Menopause

When you have sore joints and muscles, cramps or headaches, you can use this simple yet powerful process to put your pain at bay so you can enjoy your everyday activities. Of course, pain is a signal from the body and any undiagnosed pain should be reported to your medical professional.

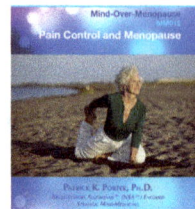

MM13 – Three Easy Steps To Regaining Balance

Many women experience irregular cycles and mood swings while transitioning into menopause. Some women may even experience sudden heart palpitations, intense anxiety or feelings of panic. Now you can find your way back to center quickly and easily. These steps, once mastered, can work for you even in the most difficult situations. With this session you will learn the three simple steps needed to regain balance in your life no matter the circumstances.

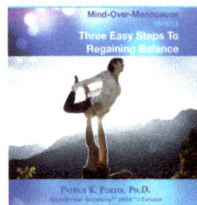

Pain-Free Lifestyle Program
Patrick K. Porter, Ph.D.

Persistent pain can have a costly impact on your life. It can lead to depression, loss of appetite, irritability, anger, loss of sleep, withdrawal from social interaction, and an inability to cope. Fortunately, with creative visualization and relaxation, pain can almost always be controlled. (CVR) helps you eliminate pain while you relax, revitalize, and rejuvenate. You deserve to be free of your pain—and now you can be, thanks to CVR!

PF01 – Tapping into a Pain-Free Lifestyle

Dr. Patrick Porter will guide you through a simple exercise to transform pain into relaxation. You'll tap into your body's innate ability to heal itself, allowing the healing process to happen while you take a relaxing mental vacation. Pain will lose all power over you as you learn to relax away your pain and enjoy your life free from discomfort.

PF02 – Activate Your Mental Pharmacy

In this dynamic process, you'll unlock your body's natural pharmacy, flushing pain from your body and neutralizing all discomfort. You will so galvanize your mind's healing capacity, all you'll have to do is say the word to release pain, fear and anxiety. Most importantly, you'll have this healing power at your fingertips—when and where you need it most.

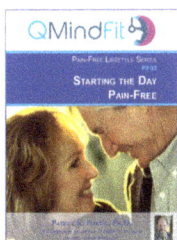

PF03 – Starting the Day Pain-Free

In this motivational session, Dr. Patrick Porter will show you that living pain-free is as simple as saying, "So-Hum;" which means transporting yourself to a pain-free state can be as easy as breathing! You'll be able to bury your pain in the past and awaken each morning pain-free.

PF04 – Developing A Pain-free Future

Dr. Patrick Porter will train you to relax deeply with this process that helps you break through the pain barrier. Discover creative ways to unleash the power of your mind to create a future where you are living a pain-free lifestyle. Learn to go to sleep with certainty that you have the skills to awaken each and every day free from discomfort.

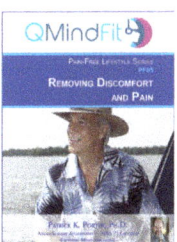

PF05 – Removing Discomfort and Pain

With this creative visualization, Dr. Patrick Porter will help you learn how positive imaging can be your key to a lifetime of relief from unwanted pain or discomfort. Let these relaxing suggestions melt your pain away as you imagine yourself in a state of optimum health and harmony for you.

PF06 – Train the Brain to Create Instant Anesthesia

Dr. Patrick Porter will train you to take these simple steps to link your body and mind so that a free flow of natural analgesia will occur even while you are awake, alert and conscious. You can use this system post-surgery, in the dental chair, or daily to remove arthritis or joint pain. Life gets exciting when you are back in control.

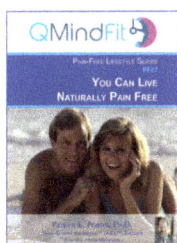

PF07 – You Can Live Naturally Pain Free

With this process, Dr. Patrick Porter provides a thorough summary of the advice and information on ho to live naturally pain free, including breathing, visualization and other relaxation techniques. Even if you are using medication, you can use the power of your mind to lessen your discomfort. You may even find that you can lessen or eliminate your need for pain medicine. *Note: Never make changes to your medication without first consulting with your doctor.*

PF08 – Erase Chronic Pain and Enjoy Life Again

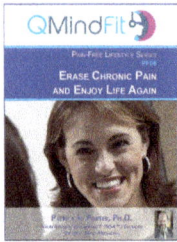

Dr. Patrick Porter uses a very compassionate, encouraging visualization process that engages kindness towards yourself and your body. He guides you to a place where you can slowly and gently make peace with your pain. The emphasis throughout this process is on letting acceptance happen, rather than trying to make it happen with your conscious mind; and his caring words and soothing voice help guide you through the process.

PF09 – Break the Emotional Bond to Physical Pain

Dr. Patrick Porter uses an advanced time-line technique to help you flex your mind's pain-reducing muscles. You will discover your own power to reduce or eliminate pain by releasing the emotional bonds you may have with your pain. Your focus will be on creating powerful, positive experiences that will, in turn, create the remarkable brain chemicals that work with your body to eliminate discomfort.

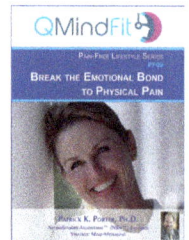

PF10 – Develop a Healthy Pain-free Attitude

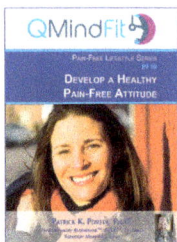

During this process, you will become aware of any resistance your body may have to becoming pain free. Even though on a conscious level you can't think of a reason for the pain, pain is a signal to the body. The pain could be physical, emotional, mental, or all three. Dr. Patrick Porter will guide you through a discovery of the faculties of your mind that release negativity and move you forward with a life-changing positive attitude about your body and mind.

PF11 – Mend Your Mind, Mend Your Body

With this relaxing process, you will use proven techniques for improving your self-esteem and assertiveness, helping you to feel better about yourself and plan your life more successfully. Dr. Patrick Porter will help you to develop a meaningful relationship between your mind and body, giving you the skills needed for a lifelong pain-free style of living.

PF12 – Develop Instant Pain Relief Triggers

It's easy to develop effective life skills when you have an arsenal of relaxation techniques and pain relief triggers. During this process, Dr. Patrick Porter will teach you useful tools for not only mastering the pain-free state, but for embracing a healthier lifestyle as well. These techniques are valuable in helping you to relieve physical discomfort regardless of whether or not you are currently in pain.

PF13 – Generate the Relaxation Response to Remove Pain

As Dr. Patrick Porter guides you to relax each part of your body, you learn to associate pain-free states in a totally new way. As you relax, you will imagine a healing sanctuary that supports relaxation and your mind's belief in your right to be healthy, strong and vibrant. In this space you feel safe and protected as you visualize healing energy filling your body.

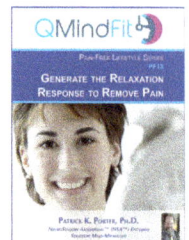

Stress-Free Childbirth

Bringing a child into the world should be an amazing life experience. Sadly, for many women, the joy of the event is lost due to fear, stress and pain. Also, research has shown that a fetus can actually feel the stress, worry, and negative emotions of the mother during pregnancy. Fortunately, with the discovery of the mind/body connection, women have an alternative—creative visualization and relaxation. This breakthrough series by Dr. Porter is designed to help the mother-to-be to relax, let go of stress, and enjoy the entire process of pregnancy, delivery and motherhood. In addition, the listener is taught to use the power of thought to create an anaesthetized feeling that can transform pain into pressure throughout labor and delivery—making the entire process stress-free for the entire family.

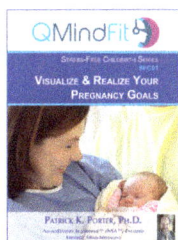

CB01 – Visualize and Realize Your Pregnancy Goals

Patrick K. Porter, Ph.D. will take you on a journey of the imagination where you'll train your brain to stay focused and on task. With this process, you'll start experiencing the relaxation response, set healthy priorities, and prepare your body for the many changes it will go through for the next nine months and beyond. This is the foundation session for the complete Stress-Free Childbirth program.

CB02 – Mental Skills for Pregnancy and Delivery

With this session negative thinking melts away and a calm state of emotional readiness replaces fear. The power of positive expectancy will lead you to positive results. Once you experience this mental training, and gain the relaxed mindset and inner confidence you need for motherhood, others may actually look to you for support!

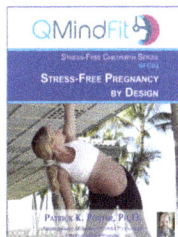

CB03 – Stress-Free Pregnancy By Design

Dr. Patrick Porter will help you learn healthy ways to manage the stress of pregnancy. In this session you'll feel your worry melt away as you experience deep relaxation. There is nothing like the joy you'll feel when you start using your mind power to create a healthy environment for your newborn and you.

CB04 – Healthy Baby / Stress-Free Lifestyle

Concentration and focus are skills you'll need to experience a natural stress-free delivery. In this process, Dr. Porter will start training you to creating that anesthetized state whenever and wherever you need it. You'll feel your confidence soaring as you look forward to putting your newfound skills to work on your delivery date.

CB05 – Emotional Readiness Mental Toughness

Relax and allow your mind to build optimistic thinking during this life transition. You need only sit back, relax and watch anxiety melt away as you focus on health and wellbeing. Soon you'll notice how your confidence is growing as your baby grows. You'll build the mental toughness to convert fear into relaxation, preparing you for a memorable stress-free delivery.

CB06 – Balancing Your Life During Pregnancy

In today's world life comes at you fast. That doesn't change during pregnancy. You still have bills, housekeeping, errands, and traffic. Learn to let go of the stress and internal conflict associated with day-to-day living. You'll gain an inner serenity as you build new life skills just as surely as you are building a new life inside of you.

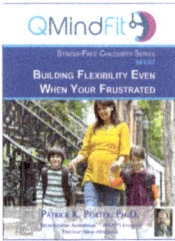

CB07 – Building Flexibility Even When Frustrated

Frustration is a given during pregnancy, and who can blame you? Your hormones are raging, your belly is swelling, and you have a dramatic life change ahead of you. With this process you'll train your body to relax and go with the flow. You'll master open and clear communication so that your entire family can be a part of your pregnancy. And, you'll focus on your health and the health of your baby.

CB08 – Building Your Delivery Team

Your mind is your best labor coach. After all, who knows what you need better than you? Now the skill of positive assertiveness can be yours. You'll know how and when to ask your family or your health care team for encouragement and support, and you'll master a breathing and relaxation technique to combat any discomfort. This process will also give you an opportunity to mentally rehearse the methods you learned in whatever birthing classes you've chosen.

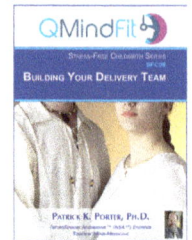

CB09 – Going With the Flow …
Transforming Contractions To Pressure

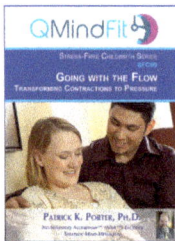

Mentally prepare yourself for the last stage of pregnancy—labor and delivery. Learn how to manage your contractions as they increase in strength and frequency so you'll remain calm and breathe properly during and between contractions. Dr. Porter will help you plan for when your contractions reach peak intensity so that, with the power of your mind, you can feel only pressure and keep your body as stress-free as possible.

CB10 – Quick Tricks For Stress-Free Delivery

By using one of Dr. Porter's favorite processes, you'll be ready to manage every aspect of your delivery. You'll focus on a safe, natural childbirth. And, best of all, with this mental exercise, you'll discover the keys to using your mind to accomplish your loftiest goals for motherhood and for life.

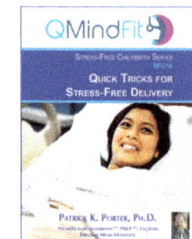

CB11 – Preparing for Motherhood

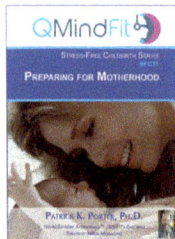

A new world awaits you after the stress-free delivery of your child. With this process, you'll be mentally, physically and emotionally prepared for motherhood. You'll discover ways to visualize solutions to problems you have not yet faced, so that even with a brand new person demanding nearly all of your attention, you can build a sense of balance back into your life.

CB12 – Enjoying Life after Pregnancy

Research shows that 20% of new moms experience postpartum depression. Dr. Porter will help you control the mood swings, anxiety, guilt, and persistent sadness that sometimes appear after childbirth. This process is to be used after the birth and can benefit a new mom for up to four months. Throughout the process you'll mentally rehearse your new lifestyle with joy and happiness for the entire family.

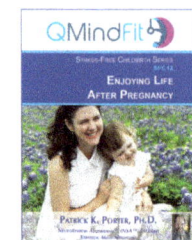

CB13 – Weight Loss and the New Mother

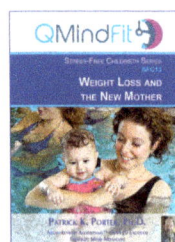

Once the new bundle has arrived and time commitments have changed, it's easy for a new mom to make her needs secondary to those of her family. You will discover easy tools to manage time and make your health and the health of your baby a top priority. Eating healthy has never been easier when you learn to use the power of your mind. Now there is no reason to hold on to that baby fat. You can lose all the weight you want naturally and healthfully.

Stress-Free Dentistry Series
Patrick K. Porter, Ph.D.

Whether you are someone who gets sweaty palms at the thought of a dentist's drill, hyperventilates the moment you lay eyes on a dental syringe, or simply gets butterflies in your stomach before going to the dentist, this program can benefit you. Studies show that over 40% of all people have a fear of dentistry. Other research demonstrates that having poor oral health can decrease your life expectancy by five years.

Fear of the dentist can have many causes, some of which are objective, and others of which are subjective. For example, if you once experienced a great deal of pain while having a tooth pulled, the next time you need an extraction, you will likely be fearful because of your previous experience. This is subjective fear. On the other hand, if you later told a friend about your bad experience, and he subsequently became fearful when faced with a tooth extraction, this would be objective fear.

Fear in and of itself is not bad. We are all born with certain fears that protect us, such as the fear of falling and the fear of loud noises. Fear stops us from doing dangerous things. The purpose of this series is to put fear in its proper perspective so that you can have a relaxed experience at every dental visit and enjoy the benefits of having healthy teeth and gums.

SFD01 – Relax and Control the Dental Experience

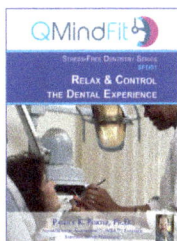

Allowing thoughts to control your emotions is a normal human experience. In this process, Dr. Patrick Porter will help you reverse this tendency, so you can control your emotions and stop reacting to negative thoughts. You will learn a simple yet powerful technique that will have you visualizing a pleasant visit to your dentist's office. You will also be guided through a process of releasing any emotions you may have tied to negative personal history experiences with dental or medical procedures

SFD02 – Mental Rehearsal for Instant Relaxation

Developing coping skills is a key element to overcoming your fear of dentistry. With this relaxing process, Dr. Patrick Porter will teach you to use a distraction technique that will eliminate anxiety and fear. Dentistry may not ever be fun for you, but it can be a relaxed and comfortable experience as you master these visualization techniques.

SFD03 – Eliminate False Beliefs & Build Self-Confidence

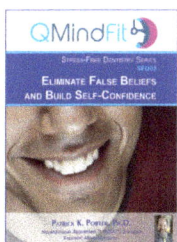

In this process you will explore beliefs about dentistry and eliminate those that are impacting you negatively. You will build the self-confidence necessary to comfortably handle any dental appointment, whether it be a cleaning, filling, or a more complex procedure. With these blocks gone, who knows? You might even enjoy your next dental experience!

SFD04 – Setting Expectations & Eliminating Dental Anxiety

Anxious reactions are natural whenever we face the unknown. In this visualization, Dr. Patrick Porter will be guiding you through processes that quickly build your self-esteem, enhance your assertiveness, and have you acting as your own advocate, asking the right questions so you understand even the most complex procedure.

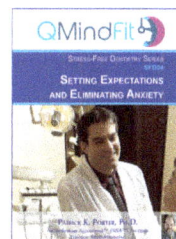

SFD05 – Control What You Think and Feel

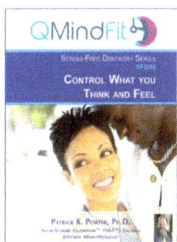

Since energy always follows thought, in this creative visualization you will master the art of singular thinking. This will allow you to create a state of relaxation where you can control the sensations in your body by controlling your thoughts. It's easier than you think to control your dental experience, and certainly worthwhile so you'll have a lifetime of healthy teeth and gums.

Vibrant Health Series
Patrick K. Porter, Ph.D.

Of all the cells in your body, more than 50,000 will die and be replaced with new cells--all in the time it took you to read this sentence! Your body is the vehicle you have been given for the journey of your life. How you treat your body determines how it will treat you. Dr. Patrick Porter, PhD will show you how, by using Q MindFit technology, you can recharge and energize your body, mind, and spirit. This series is for people who are looking for more than good health. It's for those who will settle for nothing less than vibrant health!

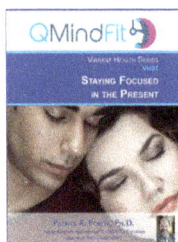

VH01 – Staying Focused in the Present

Your emotions can either help your body stay healthy, or they can be the cause of disease. Negative feelings such as regret, worry, or anxiety about an upcoming event not only waste your precious life, but also add stress to the body, which makes you more susceptible to disease. Dr. Porter will help you stay present and focused on the beauty of each moment.

VH02 – Visualize a Heart-Healthy Lifestyle

Heart disease is not a male issue alone. It is the top killer of American women. To protect your heart, you need a plan that includes movement, a healthy diet, and a positive mental attitude. You'll find smiling even easier now that you are taking an active roll in protecting the health of your heart.

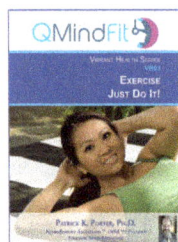

VH03 – Exercise—Just Do It!

Did you know that our human bodies recreate our skeletons every three months, we get an entirely new skin each and every month, and our bodies are brand new within two years? This means that the only thing getting older is our thoughts. Exercise is proven to help you live a longer, happier, and healthier life.

VH04 – Unlocking the Healing Force of Positive Thoughts

You are what you think about all day long. If you want to feel and look great, monitor your thoughts closely to ensure that you are thinking only positive, forward-moving thoughts. Dr. Porter will teach you a visualization technique that will help you catch negative thoughts before they can harm you and then turn those thoughts around into a positive affirmation.

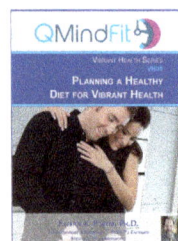

VH05 – Planning a Healthy Diet for Vibrant Health

How do you think your life would change if fresh, healthy, and live foods were the foods you craved? In this process, you will visualize a healthy lifestyle where the live foods are appealing to you, and the processed and fast foods are a big turn-off. Health care practitioners will tell you that you have to provide your physical body with high quality fuel if you want it to run properly.

VH06 – Train Your Brain to Give You Adequate Rest

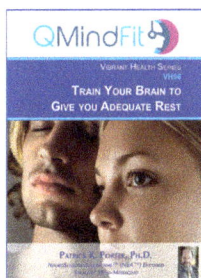

During this Q MindFit session, Dr. Porter will teach you to move through the wide-awake state of beta, into the relaxation state known as alpha, and then into the creative state known as theta. From here you will easily train your brain to provide you uninterrupted sleep. Science has shown that for sleep to be healing and rejuvenating, you need to engage the REM pattern. REM sleep is your nervous system's way of healing and refueling your body.

VH07 – Problem Solving For Vibrant Health

A sharp mind is essential to optimum brain health, and mental exercise and brain stimulation are the keys to maintaining an active mind. The brain creates unhealthy neuro-chemicals whenever you are focused on problems. By placing your attention on solutions, you encourage your brain to create the healthy neuro-chemicals that make you feel good.

VH08 – Supercharge Your Memory & Concentration

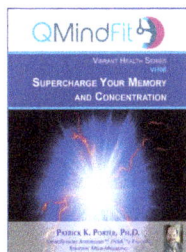

Dr. Porter will teach you simple tips for improving your everyday memory of names, addresses, events, and whatever else you wish to remember. You will gain confidence in knowing that your memory is getting stronger and your brain is staying healthy as you move through this journey we call life.

VH09 – Surround Yourself With a Great Support System

Whether family, friends or coworkers, the company you keep plays a key roll in the health of your mind and body. Dr. Porter will give you tactful ways to keep yourself surrounded from every side with positive-minded, healthy people who are on your team—people who will care for, support, love, respect, and appreciate you as you reach your goal of vibrant health.

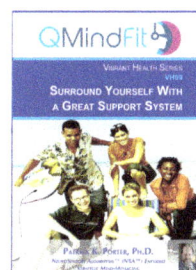

VH10 – Release Tension and Create Relaxation

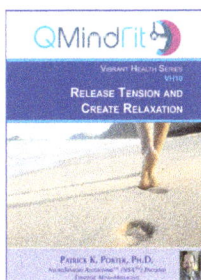

Learning relaxation techniques is a great way to help with stress management. Relaxation isn't just about peace of mind or enjoying a hobby. Relaxation is, a process that decreases the effects of stress on your mind and body. With this technique you will learn the 3 easy steps that Dr. Porter teaches his clients to transform their lives.

Accelerated Learning System
Patrick K. Porter, Ph.D.

Whether you are an honor student or just having difficulty taking a test, this breakthrough learning system will help you overcome learning challenges and accelerate your current skill level. Imagine doubling your reading speed while improving your memory. Sit back, relax and allow your mind to organize your life, while you build your self-confidence and earn better grades with Dr. Porter's complete learning system.

ALS01 – Setting Goals for Learning Success

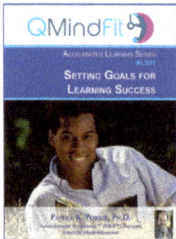

Dr. Porter's Pikeville College study proved that the more successful students are those who have an outcome or ultimate goal in mind. With this module you will learn the secrets of goal setting, experience a boost in motivation, and see your self-confidence in the classroom soar.

ALS02 – Being an Optimistic Thinker

Henry Ford once said, "Whether you think you can, or you think you can't, you are right." It all starts with attitude. You will be guided into the creative state, where you'll discover ways of breaking through to your optimistic mind that will help you to think, act and respond with a positive nature even during your most difficult classes or around challenging people.

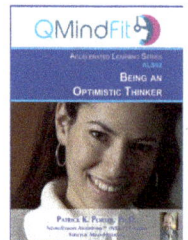

ALS03 – Six Steps to Using Your Perfect Memory

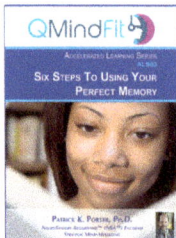

Harness the natural byproduct of relaxing your mind by using the six steps that activate a perfect memory. You will discover creative ways to access and recall the information you need as you need it! Best of all, you will have this ability the rest of your life.

ALS04 – Secrets for Increasing Your Reading Speed

Our minds absorb every word on a page as soon as we scan it. This module features ways to break through the barriers that prevent you from reading at the speed and comprehension level you desire. It's simpler and easier than you think!

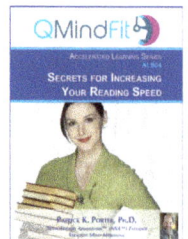

ALS05 – Using the Tricks of Highly Successful Students

With this creative process you will learn the best-kept secrets of successful students and how to apply them in your own life. You will soon discover that if someone else can do what you want to do, you can model what that person is doing and master it for yourself.

ALS06 – Problem Solving with Your Creative Mind

Imagine following in the footsteps of great thinkers such as Einstein, Edison and Chopin - all of whom used creative visualization to spark their imaginations. You will discover how to step into the realm of infinite possibility where imagination and creativity are limitless, and how to solve your everyday problems with solutions found in the present as well as the future.

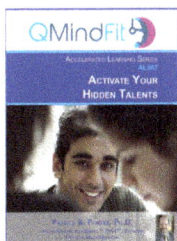

ALS07 – Activate Your Hidden Talents

Your skills and talents go beyond your one-dimensional IQ (Intelligence Quotient). In fact, there are a multitude of intelligences. Relax with this module and you will activate the different stages of intelligence within you, making you a person of intellect on multiple levels.

ALS08 – Demonstrate Self-Confidence in Learning

Concentration is key to learning. You will discover during this module a powerful concentration exercise that will unlock your true confidence. Once unlocked, you can succeed at anything you put your mind to in ways you never dreamed possible!

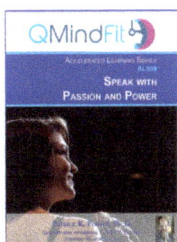

ALS09 – Speak with Passion and Power

You might not have been born a public speaker, but with these foolproof methods to activate your other-than-conscious mind, you will speak with passion on any topic. You will have the power and skill to speak freely, easily and clearly, whenever you're presenting, without stumbling or hesitation.

ALS10 – End Self-Sabotage at School

Imagine pulling out the roots of sabotage and planting the seeds of greatness that will help you in the classroom. With this specially designed module, you will eliminate old patterns that are holding you back. You will eliminate the time bandits and unleash your ultimate power to manifest your dreams in and out of the classroom.

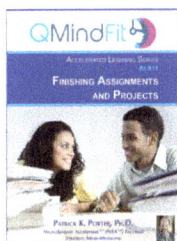

ALS11 – Finishing Assignments and Projects

Imagine tapping into the unseen power of your other-than-conscious mind to get organized and efficiently complete any project. That is exactly what you will be doing with this session as you use creative visualization and relaxation to set internal time-lines and finish projects.

ALS12 – Turning Homework Procrastination into Motivation

This module will have you practicing the eight steps to transform procrastination into motivation. You will have more fun completing your homework or starting a new project than you ever dreamed possible.

ALS13 – The Power of Affirmations in the Classroom

You will discover how the right words can create a powerful mental image of you in the classroom. Let your other-than-conscious mind quickly put into motion all the right actions that will lead you to your educational goals.

Better Life Me
Patrick K. Porter, Ph.D.

BLM01 – Committing To Your Balanced Life

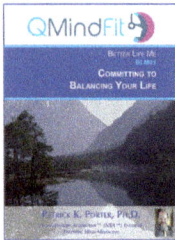

During this visualization Dr. Patrick Porter (PHD) will help you to integrate the 8 essential segments of the Wheel of Life. Your other-than-conscious will help you to create good health, incorporate strategies to build wealth and take control of your finances just to name a few. This session prepares you for the foundation of the 8 core areas of the Wheel of Life training, assisting you in living a better life now.

BLM02 – Health and Wellbeing Visualization

In this integration you will imagine the role food and drinks have in creating your better life now. Dr. Porter will have you creating a time-line for change that will have you eating and drinking the most nutritious foods available. Making that mind/body connection will help you to maintain your healthiest weight. Imagine the joy of exercise as you plan your healthy future.

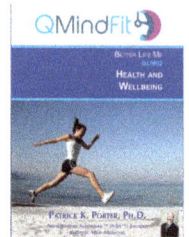

BLM03 – Wealth and Finances Visualization

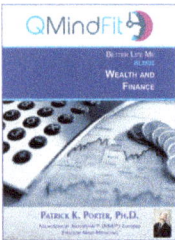

As you journey inside to the resources of your mind you will discover why wealth is a creation of your mind. Dr. Patrick Porter will show you why you managing your wealth and finances starts with the way you manage your thoughts. Learn to master your thoughts and master your finances. You learn the secrets of the wealth builders and realize why wealth can be defined as what you have left if you lose all your money; and why money is not wealth. You will visualize how to put money to work for you so that you can achieve what you want to achieve and do what you want to do.

BLM04 – Relationships Visualization

Relationships start with you. As you integrate this lesson at the other than conscious level, you will use your creative mind with your soul mate, children, mom, dad, uncles, aunts, cousins, neighbors and friends. You will visualize life not as a competition, but as a learning experience. It will be natural for you to be easy going and accepting. You will be amazed at how easy it is to let everyone have their own opinion, without wanting to WIN over them.

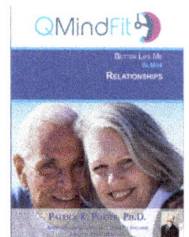

BLM05 – Lifestyle Visualization

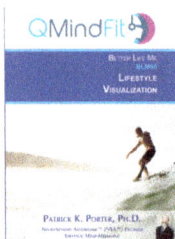

Your life will transform from the inside out as you eliminate consumerism and master the time in your life. With mass control everyone you can develop strong beliefs that will guide your behavior. During this visualization, Dr. Patrick Porter will help you work through any judgements you might have of yourself or what others think of you; and develop the simple balanced life that will bring you the greatest joy by releasing the past, embracing the present and looking forward to the future.

BLM06 – Personal Growth Visualization

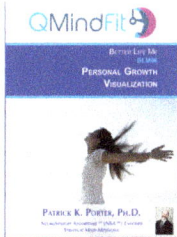

Imagine awakening your passion, and listening to your inner wisdom and exploring your life from the inside out. It is said that spirit is simple, man is complex. As Dr. Patrick Porter guides you on this mental exercise you will learn to listen to your heart. You will experience the joy of negative beliefs melting away, leaving you free to do something new. Negative emotions such as fear, frustration and anger will no longer serve you and you will no longer serve them. You will allow your guidance system to keep you on purpose and stay in touch with your passion. What would you be doing RIGHT NOW if you could do anything?

BLM07 – Career Visualization

Dr. Patrick Porter will teach you how to unlock your true potential on this guided imagery program that will work to shift your attitude so that results follow you like your shadow. You will learn how the master mentors do things at the deepest levels of the mind. You will use your strengths to draw into your world a support team that will help you get from where you are to where you want to go in the safest and quickest timeframe. Imagine what you can accomplish when you collaborate with the greatest minds around you!

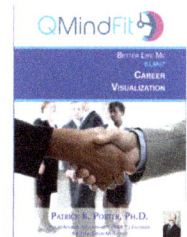

BLM08 – Environment Visualization

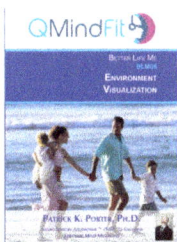

Dr. Porter will guide you through this lesson by understanding the resources you have within you. You might not be able to control the weather but you will learn to appreciate nature's gift. You will recreate your connection with the world that will empower you to take an active roll to reduce your carbon foot print and understand what the environment means to you. You will gain a new appreciate for the real value of the things nature has provided you?

BLM09 – Spirituality Visualization

During this experience, Dr. Porter will help you to understand the consciousness that is you; how as a spiritual being you are having a physical experience and how evolution in consciousness is the key to your connectivity to all things seen and unseen. You will explore your intuition and allow the happiness of your spirit to show up in your life in ways that you can't imagine with inner resources you didn't know you have.

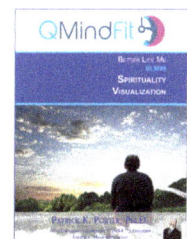

BLM10 – You Can Be The Change

You can rise above your circumstances and better yourself through personal development and self improvement. In this summary visualization, Dr. Porter using the Wheel of Life concepts, will guide you through exercises that will put your life into perspective. You will unleash the power of thought and action and strive to balance the 8 areas of your life. You will go to that quiet place within where your spirit is magnificent. It is there your determination to conquer both boundaries and limitations will drop away. You will awaken to find there is nothing stopping you from changing your life--if you let go of your limiting beliefs and exhibit the behavior and take the actions necessary to achieve the outcomes that you desire.

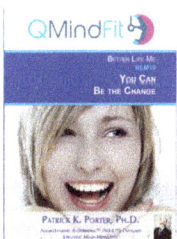

Blue Sky: Professional Airline Series

The airline industry has long been considered a "glamour" industry, but those working in the business know that once it becomes your job, you are in a constant battle to maintain the health of your body and mind. An airline professional's stress can come in many forms—from dealing with exhausting schedules and unruly passengers to the underlying fears related to travel during uncertain times. For this reason, Dr. Patrick Porter has created the Blue Sky Series, which is designed to help airline professionals regain balance in their lives through deep relaxation and creative visualization techniques delivered through its proprietary personal achievement device.

BSS1 – Sleep on Any Schedule

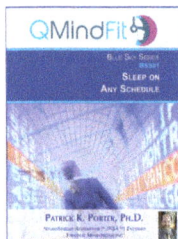

In the airline industry, flying across time zones, arriving late at night, and being expected to awaken early the next morning are all part of the job. While the occasional traveler is able to get over jet lag with relative ease, in the airline business, jet lag is part and parcel to a day's work. Unfortunately, this regular disruption of the sleep cycle can result in chronic fatigue, headaches, body aches, and a lowered immune system. Now, for the exhausted airline employee, Dr. Porter has designed a visualization technique for deep, restful, uninterrupted sleep—the kind of sleep that renews and invigorates. You will quickly discover how, through the power of your mind, you can take control of your sleep cycles for balance and good health.

BSS2 – Clear Out Flight Noise and Return to Health

With this visualization, you will be guided through some mental balancing processes to help you deal with the impact of that constant barrage of jet engine noise. During the process, you will clear your mind, reset your attention and focus on health. During this process, you will learn to de-stress, relax and have fun after a flight.

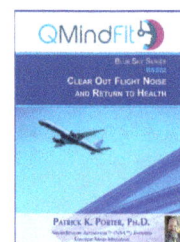

BSS3 – Planning an Optimistic Future In Flight or On the Ground

Studies have shown that as many as 80% of flight attendants are taking anti-depressants to help them cope with the stress of their jobs and related lifestyle challenges. During this visualization, Dr. Porter will guide you through a series of techniques designed to get you thinking and feeling positive about yourself, your career, and your life. The path to total wellness starts with a thought, and this session will help you focus on the thoughts that will lead to you to vibrant emotional and mental health.

BSS4 – Flight Time Eating Habits

Because of the nature of the airline industry, it is natural for you to be in a hurry most of the time. However, this doesn't have to translate to poor eating habits. Dr. Porter will be guiding you through a proven time-management visualization that will also have you setting health priorities, making good food choices as a part of your daily routine, and building a self-image for a healthy, vibrant you.

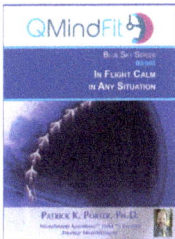

BSS5 – In Flight Calm in Any Situation\

In this powerful process, you will learn a quick and easy way to regain control of yourself physically, mentally, and emotionally, even after you have been exposed to severe turbulence or any other fear-inducing event. While others can afford to be afraid, you must be the calming, reassuring voice of reason. You will gain the confidence you need so that others will see you as a source of support during any flight situation.

BSS6 – Building Your Emotional Shield

Helping to deliver people across the country or around the world is a big responsibility. During this visualization, you will discover the healthiest way to manage this type of burden. Dr. Porter will help you to build a necessary emotional shield, even if you have a tendency to take on other people's issues and not let them go.

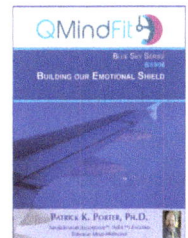

BSS7 – Removing the Stress of Emergency Situations

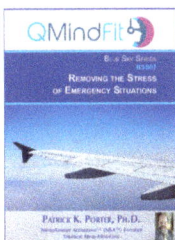

During times of high-level stress, it's normal to feel your heart rate increase, for your hands to turn cold, or for your blood pressure to rise. These reactions are all part of our built-in fight or flight response. Without a healthy way to deal with emergency situations, such as a passenger's health issues, an unruly traveler, or an emergency landing—and without the tools to deal with the post trauma of such events—it can be devastating to your physical and emotional health. During this process, you will learn how to create the relaxation response and gain the mental skills necessary to clear out these memories so that, once the crisis is over, you can return to a balanced life.

Brain Fitness Breakthrough
Patrick K. Porter, Ph.D.

Can you build a stronger brain? Patrick K. Porter, PhD believes so, and research is now verifying that regular brain stimulation and keeping the brain active helps to improve and prolong healthy brain performance. But unlike computer games that work on the conscious level and stress out the brain, Q MindFit brain stimulation creates new neural pathways and connections through the use of brainwave entrainment. These sessions are designed train the brain to stay in a state of infinite possibility and eliminate the old stuck states using the science of Neuro-Linguistic Programming (NLP). The variety, diversity and complexity of stimulation that your brain receives can make a significant difference regarding its performance. With these SMT sessions, you can have some control over what will stimulate and shape your brain and this is great news! Brain Fitness is now as easy as kicking back and taking a quick nap.

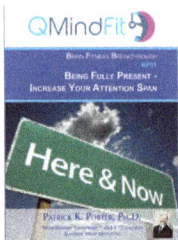

BF01 – Being Fully Present Increase Your Attention Span

In today's fast-paced, high-tech world, it's all too easy to bounce around from email to text message and back again losing focus on what's most important. During this session, Dr. Porter will guide you through the mental exercises that will have you concentrating on concepts and problems for a longer period of time. And with the use of layered Neuro-Sensory Algorithms (NSA) you will awaken from your brain entrainment session thinking more clearly and accessing skills that will improve your everyday life.

BF02 – Lighting Fast Problem Solving

In this brain fitness session, you will learn to acquire new skills faster and think more quickly, even in stressful situations. Your brain is a pattern-recognizing system and, when properly trained, can take in thousands of times the information you process consciously. Dr. Porter will guide you through a thought experiment that has been used by geniuses in the past to quickly master new skills and accelerate the learning of new information.

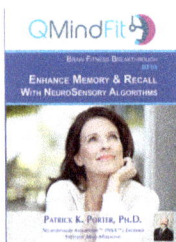

BF03 – Enhance Memory & Recall with Neuro-Sensory Algorithms

As we grow in age and wisdom, there is a social belief that we must give up our powerful memories. With this session, Dr. Patrick Porter will help you learn to organize your experiences in new and resourceful ways that will increase your intelligence and improve your recall of important information. With this type of brain training, you can keep a keen memory of facts and look forward to using your life experiences for problem solving for the rest of your life.

BF04 – Creativity Booster

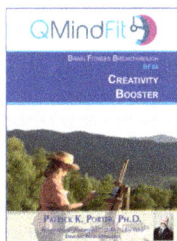

Einstein once said, "Imagination is more important than knowledge." He believed that the key to problem solving lies in your capacity to imagine. During this Brain Fitness session, Dr. Porter will guide you through specific brain entrainment frequencies for boosting Alpha, the creativity brain wave. At the same time, he while guide you through a thought experiment to supercharge your imagination. Life is about choices and effective decision-making, which comes easily when you have flexibility in your thinking. As you relax with this mental exercise, you will experience this position of power.

BF05 – Optimizing Your Brain's Capacity

Each brain entrainment session is designed to build mental flexibility and reduce stress. As you retrain your brain, organizational skills will improve, bringing you a feeling of confidence and self-control. As you stimulate creativity, focus and concentration, you will find the things that you have done well in the past improving and those mental skills that need improvement sharpening.

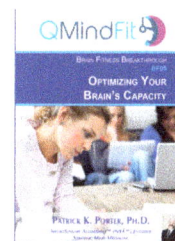

BF06 – Maintaining Focus & Concentration

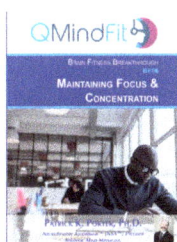

As we grow with age and maturity, there is an outdated belief that our focus becomes impaired. With this brain fitness process, you will eliminate this and other negative beliefs and build optimism about your brains capacity to stay sharp. Being more alert is a natural part of maintaining a young brain.

BF07 – Achieving Peak Performance

At times we all experience moments of peak performance. During this brain fitness session, you will capture that magical feeling and recall those mental states of clarity so that when you need those emotions and skills, you can recall and use them. The real beauty of brain fitness is that with each listening you are building new neural pathways that are staying youthful and active. You will discover that it is possible for you to have lightning fast problem-solving skills and maintain the highest level of cognitive functioning.

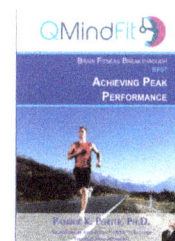

Finding Love and Building Winning Relationships
Patrick K. Porter, Ph.D.
& Michael Irving, Ph.D.

Winning at dating involves building relationship skills that you can apply to the world of dating and romance. With Dr. Michael Irving's powerful techniques, and Dr. Patrick Porter's guiding voice, this program provides you a step-by-step plan for creating a winning attitude and positive outlook, the key life skills needed to succeed at dating and in romantic relationships. Dr. Porter & Dr. Irving understand that finding a date is never easy, but you can increase your odds dramatically by harnessing the right attitude, developing the habit of positive self-talk, and changing any negative beliefs you have created around dating. This program is designed to assist you in developing the positive attitude and success-driven belief system that can make you a winner at dating and relationships.

WR00 – 10-Minute Preview Session: Building Winning Relationships

Relax with this introductory session to awaken your other-than-conscious mind to the myriad of dating possibilities before you. This session is designed to help you awaken the self-confidence within you so you can start feeling comfortable and secure in responding to the dating opportunities presented to you.

WR01 – Taking Charge of Your Dating Success

In this session, you will see how the dating game is at your door just waiting for you to embrace it. You will see yourself walking through that door with joy in your heart and a spring in your step. As you take charge of your personal approach to dating, you will find yourself trying new things to look and feel better. Taking more interest in your clothing, hair, and grooming will become second nature to you. Whether your interest in dating is about building a relationship or just having fun, you will rehearse presenting your desires honestly and openly. From that deep inner place in your mind, you develop a natural ability to socialize comfortably. Spending time with like-minded people will become natural to you.

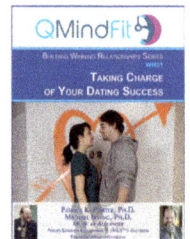

WR02 – Overcoming Shyness

We all have some form of shyness inside that's driven by the fear of rejection. This session will help you eliminate the shyness that inhibits or even paralyzes you from taking up new relationships. The inspiring words in this session will serve to transform your shyness into the confidence that you deserve to radiate. You will create a new you with radiant self-confidence. Your self-assured smile, your interest, your openness, and the confidence you exude will work together in helping you strike up conversations and hold the attention of others.

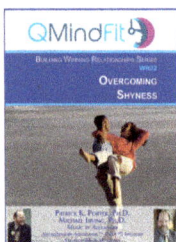

WR03 – Freedom From Criticism ... It's In Your Power

It may seem as if you have spent your entire life trying to make others happy, but this is not how you started your life journey. As a toddler, you were okay with just being you. You were a gift to life in every way that is you. Later, when others treated you with negativity, you learned to protect yourself. But the truth is, people were really trying to make up for their own feelings of low self-worth and of not being good enough. You no longer have to internalize other people's insecurities or not-good-enough belief systems. During this session, you will acquire resiliency and learn to rise above criticism at work, home, or in the activities you undertake. Your other-than-conscious mind knows you are perfectly fine just as you are. When you know you are good enough for yourself, you are naturally good enough for others.

WR04 – Increase Your Attraction Through Confident Flirting

The art of flirting is a two way dance. The confidence you display is the strongest factor in how your flirting is received. After listening to this process, you will feel confident knowing that successful flirting is a natural response. You will see yourself having fun flirting, as you comfortably send signals that you are interested and available. You will see yourself smiling, touching, and being playful as you give another person your full attention. In the two-way dance of flirting, you will learn to trust your intuition and other-than-conscious mind to know when the signs of flirting are coming your way. In fact, you will visualize yourself at a dance with a friend who is going to practice the art of flirting with you, allowing you to notice body language and the subtle nuances of flirting.

WR05 – Letting Go of Fear and Visualizing Dating Success

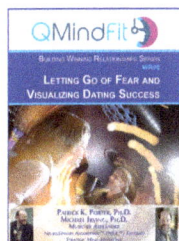

In this session, you are going to visualize a successful date as the new you who enjoys simple, casual, carefree, and fun experiences. You will visualize yourself fully prepared to go on a date with someone you like and who likes you. All hints of nervousness or anxiety have been put to rest. The smile in your eyes says you are glad to be there and you appreciate the person with whom you are sharing the moment. With both your conscious and other-than-conscious mind, you are going to feel and experience a date that turns out the way that you want. Through repeated use of this session, you will notice how each day your confidence and positive expectations of dating get better and the actions you take to improve your world become easier and more natural.

WR06 – Finding a Date In The Expansive World Around You

With this session you will learn to integrate looking for dates into your everyday social routine. During this visualization, you discover that you do not need to be pushy, obsessive or aggressive, but you also know that there are opportunities just waiting to present a special someone in your life. You will learn the art of optimism. Connecting with people suitable for dating has never been easier. You find your positive attitude is making it easier every day. You never know when an exciting and adventurous door will open for you. Any negative beliefs about dating will drift away and be replaced with a carefree, positive and confident attitude.

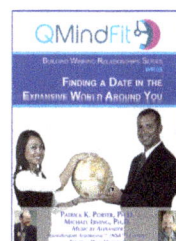

Stress Reduction Series

Stress is the most pervasive malady of our time. The effects on our health, productivity and quality of life are more devastating than most people care to admit. Luckily, you've just found the solution! Q MindFit can help you see yourself as the healthy, happy, optimistic person you'd prefer to be. With this new image, your fears and frustrations fade away, your anxiety vanishes, and you no longer let small things stress you.

SR01 – Create Your Enchanted Forest for Stress Reduction

Follow along as Dr. Patrick Porter guides you through your personal enchanted forest—a quiet, serene place where you have nothing to do but relax. Your other-than-conscious mind will massage away all tension, allowing you to release all negative thoughts and feelings. You'll return from your magical forest filled with positive feelings, able to enjoy and express your true inner peace.

SR02 – Create Your Mountaintop Retreat for Stress Reduction

Say goodbye to all stress and confusion as you take a trip to this breathtaking mountaintop retreat. When you listen to this restful process, using your mind to relax your body will become as comfortable and automatic as breathing. The stress, strain and confusion of everyday life will melt away as you awake refreshed, revitalized and renewed!

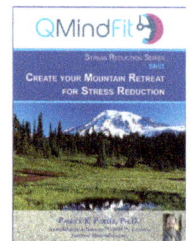

SR03 – Experience Dream-time and Achieve Your Goals

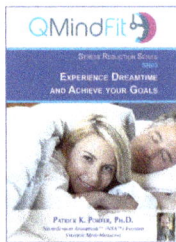

Possibilities are limitless in your dreams! In this CVR session by Dr. Patrick Porter, you'll walk along your dream beach, leaving behind all stress, worry and tension. During your dreamtime, you'll be able to change past failures into triumphs—even meet your future self to see the successes you've achieved. You'll use your dreams to develop hidden talents, skills and abilities, and awaken convinced that infinite success will be yours.

SR04 – Putting Future Events Into Perspective

Research has proven that 97% of what we worry about never happens in the way we fear. With this powerful visualization, Dr. Patrick Porter will show you the benefits of having a healthy picture of the future. You will be amazed by what you can do when you learn to magnify positive thoughts. You'll put your future into perspective and learn creative ways to live your life without unhealthy stress. Your future will become bright and compelling as you take an active part in planning your personal success.

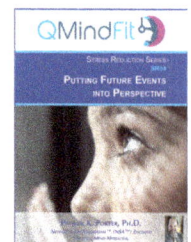

SR05 – Reducing Uncertainty And Doubt

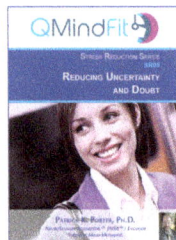

When you cast out doubt, all that can remain is the truth—and the truth is you are more capable than you have been led to believe. Dr. Patrick Porter will guide you on the road to discovering hidden talents that will help you reduce or eliminate doubt. Just as a sponge absorbs water, so too your mind will soak up these soothing visualizations and train your brain to yield spontaneous relaxation, helping you to create a dynamically healthy body.

SR06 – Eliminating Negative Thinking

Research has proven that negative thinking has a chemically negative effect on the body. With this visualization, Dr. Patrick Porter will help you to experience the healing force of your mind. Once your own healing power is working within your body, you will build a shield of protection against anything that is less than vibrant health for you. It will become second nature to eliminate negative thoughts as you enjoy the energy of positive thoughts and actions.

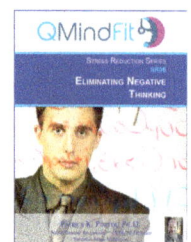

SR07 – Making Peace With Your Past

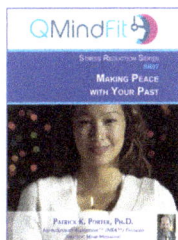

Your past works as a filter helping you make decisions about the present and the future. When you release the emotional baggage that is holding you back from a true commitment to healthy living, attaining optimum health becomes easy. Dr. Patrick Porter will teach you to forgive, forget, and move on with a healthy body and attitude. With the power of forgiveness on your side, the unseen forces of your mind will go to work creating radiant health.

SR08 – Rehearse Mental Harmony for Physical Health

Dr. Porter will guide you through mental rehearsal for setting and accomplishing your health goals. With this powerful process you will actively use mental housecleaning techniques to cleanse your mind of negative beliefs from your past, and then help you to unleash your body's natural ability to create perfect health.

SR09 – Stress-free Mind, Healthy Body

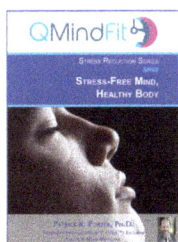

You will enjoy learning how everything starts with a thought and then becomes a thing. In much the same way as your shadow reflects your physical form, your thoughts, actions and beliefs shape your body. Sit back, relax and enjoy discovering these amazing secrets for cultivating a healthy mind and enjoying life in a dynamically healthy, strong body.

SR10 – Developing Spontaneous Relaxation

Sometimes you need to relax and get focused right now! During this session, Dr. Patrick Porter will train your other-than-conscious mind to soak up a series of soothing creative visualization and relaxation processes, and train your brain to yield relaxed and positive thoughts on demand.

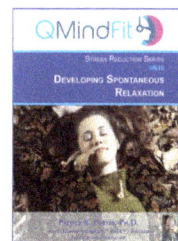

SR11 – Free Your Mind & Experience Your Healthy Body

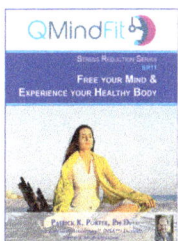

We think thousands of thoughts every day. Learn how to cast out the negative, listen to the positive, and unleash your mind's healing force. You will build a shield of protection against anything that might stop you from experiencing radiant good health.

SR12 – Creating a Life of Vibrant Health

You will learn how easy it is to release any hurts from your past that might holding you back from your commitment to health. This process engages the healing graces that allow you to forgive, forget, and move on with a healthy body and attitude.

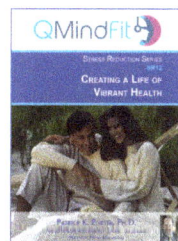

SR13 – Allowing a Life of Health & Abundance

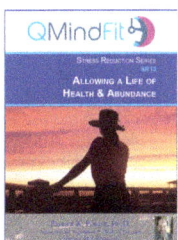

Some people think they need stress to be motivated. In this session, you will learn to use positive motivators to get what you want. You will be guided through the garden in your mind where you will train your other-than-conscious to focus on action, success, and health. Working with the healing intelligence of the body has never been easier as you learn new and creative ways to live your life without the need for stress.

10 Min AM Sessions

The Q MindFit light and sound technology must be experienced to be understood. In Dr. Patrick Porter's own words, "Trying to tell someone what it's like to experience the system is like trying to describe atmosphere to a fish." In this ten-minute demo, you will be introduced to the four major brainwave frequencies and find out how the Q MindFit guides you to the two most beneficial of them. You will even practice using visualization and will experience a mental vacation to your personal place of relaxation. Once you have completed the session, we're sure you'll agree that learning to use your mind is one of the most powerful steps you can take toward improving your life.

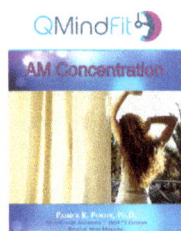

AM Concentration

This session has been designed to boost your self-esteem. A key benefit of creative visualization and relaxation is to help you improve your self belief. With this morning program, taking ten minutes to visualize your daily goals, while at the same time enjoying greater focus and concentration.

AM Focus

Dr. Porter has designed this process to provide the mental clarity necessary to begin the day with focus. Our lives are typically filled with distractions, and spending these ten short minutes upon awaking is a great way help put ourselves in the proper mind-set to easily deal with such distractions, while staying on course to achieve our objectives for the day.

AM Motivation

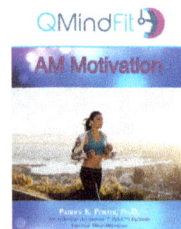

Today is the day you can take back control of your feelings so you can enjoy greater focus and concentration and that means the motivation to get things done. With this 10 minute motivation session, you will change procrastination into that confident person you desire to be. Each of the AM programs are designed to help you become successful and enjoy greater focus and concentration.

20 Min PM Sessions
PM Creating Your Success Time-line

Imagine drifting off into a deeply rejuvenating sleep while the most powerful computer on earth continues to plan a time-line for success. That is exactly what Dr. Porter has created in this program. You will be guided into restful sleep while your powerful mind plans success in your daily life.

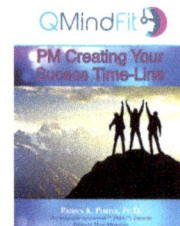

PM Focus In Dreamtime

Sleep often eludes us when our minds are cluttered with leftovers from the day's events. Dr. Porter created this program to help us enter into the deepest level of sleep by putting today's activities into perspective.

PM Release Negativity

With this session you will train the brain to shut off the stress and negativity of the day and drift off into a deeply relaxing state of sleep where you focus on the positive and eliminate the negative. The results will have you awakening with more energy and motivation to accomplish any task during the following day.

ZenSync Meditations

Ancient wisdom tells us that "our needs are few and our wants are many." At time you might want to just contemplate with the alpha music and the light and sound technology guiding you into that "Zen" state of mind. Whether you have 10 minutes or 25 we have provided you with conscious choices, and free thinking in a consumer-driven world to create your own mental vacation.

The Blue Chip Mind of Championship Basketball
With Anthony Simms & Patrick K. Porter, Ph.D.

There are two kinds of motivation that enable basketball players to achieve greatness. The first type is extrinsic motivation that comes from external influences such as coaches and peers. Athletes are extrinsically motivated to earn awards and social recognition. The second kind is intrinsic motivation, an inherent characteristic that feeds off one's inner drive to accomplish a goal.

After former Olympian and NBA player Anthony Simms experienced Dr. Patrick Porter's Creative Visualization/ Relaxation techniques, he recognized it as a way for the youths he mentors to build the intrinsic motivation and commitment of a champion. He saw Q MindFit as a solution for the many young competitors who could never afford a personal sports psychologist, and as a way for athletes to easily practice mental rehearsal, a proven method for improving skills and instilling muscle memory.

BCB00 – Demo: Communication of Champions

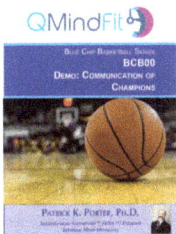

Anthony's experience as a New York Knick gave him a unique perspective on athletic communication. With Anthony's guidance, Dr. Porter designed this program to help you experience the benefits of the Q MindFit by using the communication skills of champions. To demonstrate the power of your mind, he will guide you through a visualization for staying in the moment and a technique for alerting your teammates of your opponent's noticeable patterns. Give Anthony and Dr. Porter ten minutes and they will show you how to unleash your excellence on the court.

BCB01 – Developing the High Values of a Champion

As an Olympic athlete and professional player, Anthony found that the values you have in life are the values you bring to the court. Dr. Porter will help you keep your highest values present so you stay focused and motivated. During this visualization you will be called on to reach inside to that place that makes you more. Once you see it in your mind's eye, you can experience it on the court.

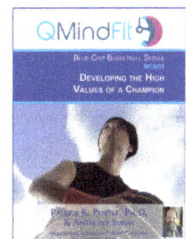

BCB02 – Reading your Opponent For Championship Play

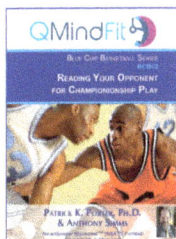

Anthony says that in a split second you need to recognize whether the player is tall or short, left- or right-handed, fast or slow, a power or finesse player, tough or soft. During this mental training you will practice a breakthrough technique called modeling. You will set up an unconscious and automatic mental program for identifying the strengths and weaknesses of your opponents, giving you a distinct advantage on the court.

BCB03 – Developing the Pre-Game Mind of a Champion

Have you ever wondered what goes through the mind of an NBA player? Anthony shares what he calls the "pre-game mind," or the ability to read your opponent's strengths and weaknesses and then go into battle mode. Dr. Porter has put this system into mental drills that will have you thinking positively and focus your energy toward success before you ever step on the court. The pre-game mind is a mental exercise and in it you are the superhero.

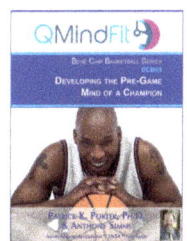

BCB04 – Developing the Post-Game Mind of a Champion

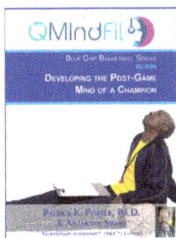

One of the biggest differences between an athlete and a champion is the "post-game mind," or the time of reflection and analysis. Dr. Porter put together a program that will provide you with the skills needed to review your performance with no regrets or judgments. The post-game mind puts you into a state of preparedness for your next game and your daily routine. The post-game mind recalls and celebrates both your brilliant plays and your small accomplishments.

BCB05 – Using the Science of Observation to Create Your Winning Skills

You can greatly improve your edge by understanding the dynamics of basketball movement, rotation, and direction. With Anthony's guidance, Dr. Porter created this session to help you master your understanding of rotation, arch, precision entry through the rim, and motion of release. Now when you watch great shooters, you will be in the habit of building your basketball IQ.

Sports/Athletic Performance

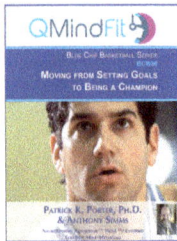

BCB06 – Moving from Setting Goals and Dreaming to Being a Champion

When Anthony is asked what one final word a champion truly understands, that word is commitment. With mental practice comes physical excellence. You will develop the clarity about what you want to do and then you will get into a mode of making it happen. Dr. Porter will help you ignite a burning desire and an all-out laser focus on your championship goals.

BCB07 – Moving from a Novice to a Champion with Lightning Speed

While novices focus on one aspect of their talent, champions know they must transform weaknesses into strengths. Time spent listening to this session is time spent mastering the skills of a champion from the inside out. If you learn poorly, you perform poorly; when you learn correctly, through the mind's eye, almost anything is achievable.

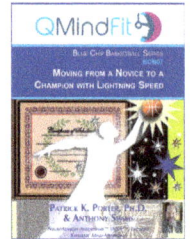

BCB08– Understanding the Metaphysics of Basketball

That which separates good athletes from champions is something beyond the physical. During this session, Dr. Porter will help you find that inner place where you move faster, jump higher, and meet the rim with ease. As you progress through this visualization, you will see yourself delivering offensive and defensive actions effortlessly. This skill will allow you to perform on the court with a disciplined edge that your opponents will never see coming.

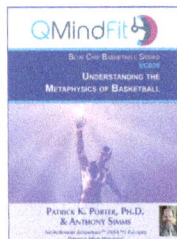

BCB09 – Blue Chip Basketball

This session focuses on the mindset of the elite, blue chip athletes who repeatedly think: "I do the most productive thing at every given moment to achieve excellence." These mental exercises are to help you identify with these blue chip athletes who aspire to perform at their optimum level on and off the court each and every day. Anthony says that every athlete has brilliance inside, and with this visualization you will learn to bring radiance into your life and game.

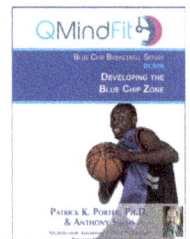

BCB10 – Standing on the Shoulders of Champions

In this session, you will apply the science of observation. While mentally hanging out with champions, you will learn to duplicate their winning advantage. You will find yourself playing with older, more mature, and more experienced players to accelerate your decision-making and performance. You will be drawn to great coaches and absorb their philosophies and techniques. In internalizing and striving for greatness, you will find yourself humble while at the same time burning with the desire to be a champion.

BCB11 – Commanding the Emotional Game of Basketball

Aggression, intensity, and self-control are words used to describe champions. These mental exercises will have you in command of yourself and your opponent at all times. You will become both focused and aggressive as you play. In aggressive, intense, and controlled play, your mind's thoughts are congruent with your physical actions and your skill of anticipatory thinking will alert you to what is going to happen moments ahead of the action.

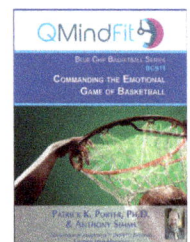

BCB12 – Developing Your Coachable Mind

A champion understands that being open to new information is key to success. Anthony calls this being coachable. In this session, you will practice mental exercises to help you keep an open mind. You will let new information empower you. Your new, coachable mind will be hungry for the information that will continually raise your level of skill and achievement. Your coachable mindset consists of not only being able to stay mentally hungry and alert, but also having the ability to learn from the different skill sets that yield success.

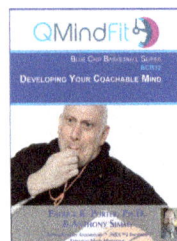

BCB13 – Activating Laser Focus

Focus is the laser-like appreciation of the next task to be accomplished. Dr. Porter will teach to have laser-like focus so you stay in the zone and everything works. You will practice focus in a new way and will develop your own activities that trigger the focus response. Focus allows your conscious competence to advance to unconscious competence—the place where the zone is your automatic state of being.

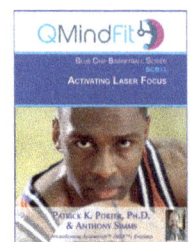

Mental Coaching For Golf
Patrick K. Porter, Ph.D.

Efficient golfers know how to relax and let their minds take over. Now, thanks to these creative visualization and relaxation (CVR) processes, you'll learn to see yourself as a calm, confident golfer. You deserve to take pleasure in your time on the course. Thanks to the Q MindFit, you'll finally be able to let go of frustration and focus on every stroke—meaning you'll not only play better, but you'll also enjoy the game more than ever!

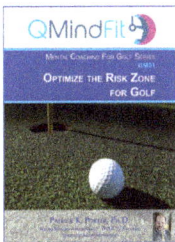

GF01 – Optimize the Risk Zone for Golf

You've never experienced a practice session like this one! Follow along with Dr. Patrick Porter as he guides you onto the driving range in your mind. Once there, you'll practice each swing, letting go of negative thoughts and allowing the clubs to do what they were designed to do—send the ball straight to the target. From now on, you'll address each ball knowing with certainty that you can see the perfect shot in your mind and achieve it in your actions.

GF02 – Develop the Attitude of a Champion

Champions understand that good outcomes come from good shots. With this dynamic process, you'll find it easy to think positive thoughts and accept each shot as it comes. You'll no longer spend time feeling distracted, over-analyzing your game, blaming the conditions of the course, or getting angry over a bad lie. Instead, you'll admire the trajectory of a well-struck drive, a clean chip shot, or a perfectly sunk putt, as you play and think like a champion!

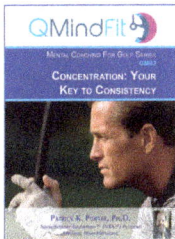

GF03 – Concentration: Your Key To Consistency

Most golf professionals consider concentration to be the key to playing golf… but almost no one teaches it. In this energizing process by Dr. Patrick Porter, he'll teach you to achieve the concentration you need simply by sitting back, relaxing, and letting go of all stress and confusion. You'll learn to block out distractions, focus like never before, and discover the concentration that will help you play the best golf of your life!

GF04 – Discover the Confidence of a Tiger

Even golfing greats get nervous when their game is on the line. Now you can sit back and relax with this revitalizing session while you learn to face any part of the course with complete self-assurance. You have good instincts—you just have to trust them! From now on you will, as you awaken ready to use the positive power of your mind--while your golfing buddies marvel at your newfound confidence.

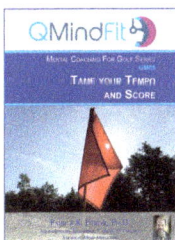

GF05 – Tame Your Tempo and Score

Because the average swing lasts less than two seconds, there's no time to make corrections on the course. That's why it's important to maintain a tempo during your game. Now you can sit back, relax, and let this refreshing session instill the skills you need to look at your game from the outside in, set your perfect tempo, lower your score and, most importantly, enjoy your game to the fullest.

GF06 – Rehearse Excellence and Eliminate Execution Errors

On the golf course your imagination can be your most powerful ally or your worst enemy. With this invigorating session by Dr. Patrick Porter, you'll learn to visualize the ideal shot each and every time you address the ball. Once you imagine the feeling of accomplishment you get from making all the right choices at the tee, you'll be able to stand back and enjoy your perfectly executed drive!

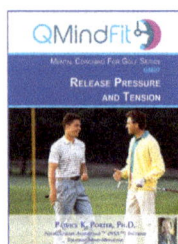

GF07 – Release Pressure and Tension

Tension is normal under certain circumstances—such as during a match—but it can also ruin your game. Thanks to this stimulating session, you'll be able to release pressure and tension under any circumstances. Loosen up, take a deep breath, and let the pressure roll away as you experience your ultimate relaxation both on and off the course.

GF08 – Gain Finesse and Lower Your Score

When you step up to the tee box expecting to win, you unleash the power of your mind to plan and produce the perfect round of golf. Research shows the mind doesn't know the difference between real and imagined. Dr. Patrick Porter will teach you techniques that will prove to you how five minutes of visualization can be equal to two hours of physical practice! With this mental edge you will have more fun on the course than ever before.

GF09 – Golf is a Mind Game... Play It!

Have you ever wondered what's in the mind of the world's greatest golfers? With this powerful modeling technique, you will be imagining what it's like to take a ride inside the mind of the golfers you most admire. Can you imagine the strokes you will shave off your score as you take advantage of his or her years of golf mastery? With this visualization you will be guided into the realm of infinite possibility where you can master each and every phase of the game you love.

GF10 – Master the Course, Master Your Round

Hitting the longest drive or sinking the unsinkable putt might be fun, but it doesn't always equal victories or low scores. Golf is a mind game you play against yourself. By learning how to play within yourself, knowing your strengths and weaknesses, you will learn to master the game. Now you can immediately improve your handicap by playing smarter and staying in control... even in the most challenging situations.

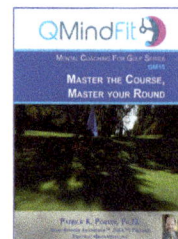

GF11 – Erase Nervousness and Perform Under Pressure

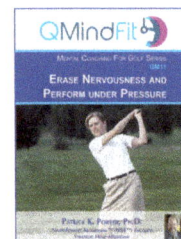

Dr. Patrick Porter will show you how a positive mental attitude will help to reduce nervousness and naturally reduce your score. Relaxation tips will help you release any anger or frustration before you address the ball. This unique visualization process will help you to regain your poise and concentration and, most importantly, control your game. Performing on the big, green stage is a breeze when you harness the power of your mind!

GF12 – Three Easy Steps to Great Golf in Any Situation

Putting together a great game is all about routine. In this insightful visualization Dr. Patrick Porter takes you from a good stance to a polished mental attitude and beyond. You'll use these keys to lower your score and enjoy it more as you open your mind to the possibilities. Consistency is key to low scores, and you'll be amazed at how easy and natural it is as you relax and rehearse the fundamentals.

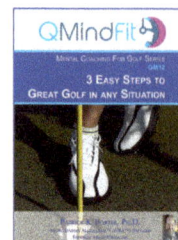

GF13 – Golfing in Dream Time... Your Key to the Ultimate Swing

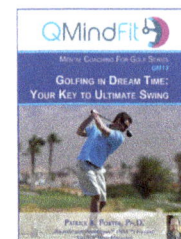

Imagine using the techniques of great inventors like Edison, Einstein and Michelangelo. That's exactly what you will be doing when Dr. Patrick Porter guides you through this powerful and fun visualization. It's been said that what the mind can conceive and believe the body will achieve. This visualization is your personal guide—from hopes and wishes to power and believability. It all starts with mentally rehearsing your goals so the unseen forces of the mind will bring them into reality!

SportZone™ Series
Patrick K. Porter, Ph.D.

Success in sports is about being the best you can be, and visualization plays a key role in getting there. Why is visualization so important? Because you get what you rehearse in life, but that's not always what you want or intend. This is especially true when you are facing the pressures of athletics. The SportZone program is designed to help you tap into the mind's potential and make your sport of choice fun and enjoyable while taking your game to the next level. Visualization for sports performance is nothing new to top competitors—athletes from Tiger Woods to diver Greg Louganis and a variety of Olympians have used visualization to bring about optimal performance, overcome self-doubt, and give themselves a seemingly unfair advantage over their competition. Now the SportZone series can work for any athlete, from junior competitors to weekend enthusiasts. Yes, you can get more out of your sport and, in the process, get more out of life.

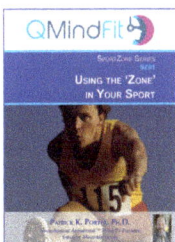

SZ01 – Using the "Zone" in Your Sport
When competitive athletes slip into their "zone" everything seems to work just right. Dr. Patrick Porter will help you get to that place where everything comes together. With this process you'll learn to put yourself into a state of "flow," your own personal "zone," so you can stay on top of your game. The "zone" is as easy to access as a deep breath once you have mastered the mental keys.

SZ02 – Control Your Emotions and Master Your Sport
It has been said that he or she who angers you conquers you; this is true even if the person who angers you is you! With this process you will learn a powerful self-visualization technique for keeping your emotions under control. With this easy technique you will no longer be giving away your power to others and will stop letting anger and frustration get the better of you.

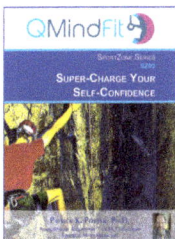

SZ03 – Super-Charge Your Self-Confidence
What would happen if you could cast out all doubt about your success? You would no longer hope, or believe, or wish it to be so—you would know it to be so! What if you could rid yourself of all doubt by simply changing your personal history (or at least your perception of it) and developing positive self-talk? You would super-charge your self-confidence, right? Well, that is exactly what you will learn with this process.

SZ04 – Psych Yourself Up! – and Perform Your Best Under Pressure
With this session Dr. Porter will help you to gain the courage to win. This may sound simple but what separates the best from the rest is mental toughness. You will be given the specific step-by-step strategies you need to perform your best under pressure now. Your success starts by eliminating "outcome anxiety" and ends with your willingness to visualize success.

Sports/Athletic Performance

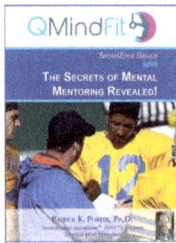

SZ05 – The Secrets of Mental Mentoring Revealed!

Everyone has an inner champion. With this breakthrough technique you will awaken yours and train it to go to work for you round the clock. Soon your other-than-conscious mind will be finding solutions and achieving goals even while you work, play, and sleep!

SZ06 – Set Goals Like the Pros

In this process Dr. Patrick Porter teaches you the secrets of full-sensory goal setting. You will develop the concentration to focus on daily, weekly and monthly goals and develop such self-discipline that others will be amazed at your determination.

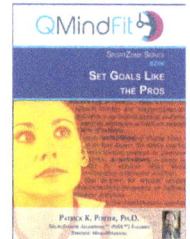

SZ07 – Feel the Pressure and Win!

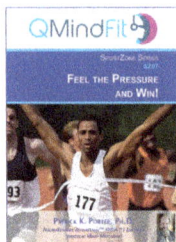

Whether you perform well under pressure or not, in this process Dr. Patrick Porter will help you learn ways to transform negative pressure into an iron will. Your other-than-conscious will then use that newfound inner strength to create results for you in sports and in life. Imagine how your body will respond when you train your brain to cast out doubt and step into the "zone" where success comes to you easily.

SZ08 – Build Desire, Drive & Perseverance

In this process you will learn how to create a compelling future and then draw that future to you like a powerful magnet. You will mentally train yourself to generate resources where and when you need them the most whether it's on the tee-box, a tennis court, a football field, or in your own backyard.

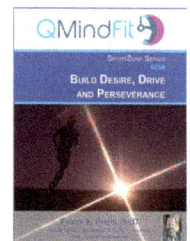

SZ09 – Think Like a Champion

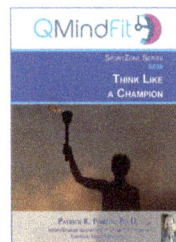

Have you ever wondered how champions think? What goes through their minds just before a game-winning field goal or a high stakes putt? In this process Dr. Patrick Porter will reveal all the leadership skills of a professional athlete so you, too, can have the confidence and determination you need when you need it the most.

SZ10 – Lessons in Sports, Lessons in Life

Dr. Patrick Porter will help you design your own creativity generator. You will build problem-solving skills, work through specific scenarios, and see yourself achieving every one of your life goals. You will use the mental toughness developed in your sport to gain that same edge in your personal life.

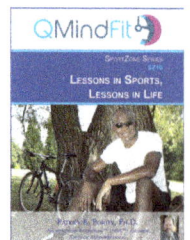

Patrick K. Porter, Ph.D. - Audio Session Catalog

Wealth Consciousness Series
Patrick K. Porter, Ph.D.

Inspired by the principles of Napoleon Hill's Think and Grow Rich.
"Imagination is the workshop of your mind, capable of
turning mind energy into accomplishment and wealth." – Napoleon Hill

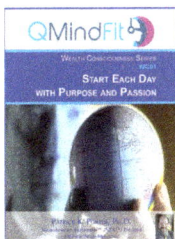

WC01 – Start Each Day with Purpose and Passion

Successful people have what Napoleon Hill called "mind energy," on their side. Dr. Patrick Porter will guide you in using this power of intention to focus your imagination on the success and prosperity you desire.

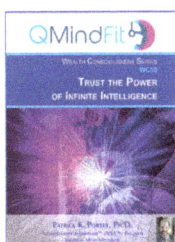

WC02 – Commit to a Life Spent with Like-Minded People

Together with Dr. Patrick Porter, you will activate what Napoleon Hill termed the "third mind," or group intelligence. With each visit to this level of the mind, your mastermind alignment will grow stronger.

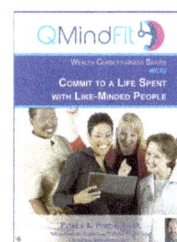

WC03 – Trust the Power of Infinite Intelligence

Do you sometimes feel as though fear of poverty has control over you? During this Q MindFit session, you will visualize and realize the thoughts and actions that bring wealth and riches into your life.

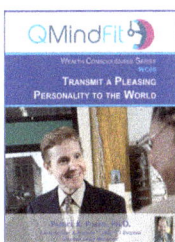

WC04 – Exceed Expectations—Serve Others, Serve Yourself

Imagine awakening each day aware that every seed you sow will come back to you as overwhelming abundance. In this session, you will become motivated by a help others mind-set. This feeling of service will magnetize wealth and abundance to you.

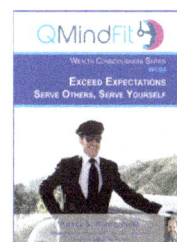

WC05 – Transmit a Pleasing Personality to the World

How might other people respond to you if you radiated enthusiasm? During this creative-visualization process, the radiant light that is your true personality will be invited out for all to see. It's easy to draw wealth and abundance to you when you show up with a pleasing personality.

WC06 – Harness The Power Of Personal Initiative

Self-motivated people tend to be the happiest and most successful. Starting the very first time you listen to this creative-visualization process, you will gain the behaviors of a self-starter. Each morning a newfound personal initiative will inspire you to greater success.

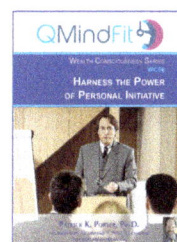

WC07 – Claim Your Right To A Positive Mental Attitude

The greatest riches in the world come from the heart. From your heart you will uncover the positive attitude that resides in that place where you dream. You will eliminate unproductive thoughts, enhance your relationships, balance your life, and make your dreams come true

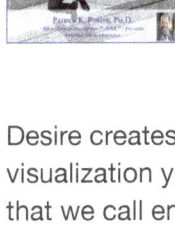

WC08 – Radiate Enthusiasm—
Your Key To Success Consciousness

Desire creates enthusiasm, which fuels determination and leads to success. During this visualization you will tap your "pulsating desire" to win—that wellspring of physical energy that we call enthusiasm.

Wearth

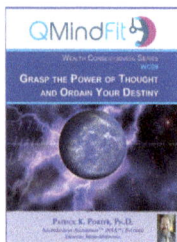

WC09 – Grasp the Power of Thought
and Ordain Your Destiny

In this visualization you will harness self-discipline, which Napoleon Hill called, "taking possession of one's mind." This new habit will stoke the inner fire that ordains your destiny. Get ready to take charge of your life as your positive new thoughts create a new world around you.

WC10 – Tune Into Infinite
Intelligence for Accurate Thinking

During this visualization, you will learn to trust your connection with infinite intelligence just as other accurate thinkers do—by thinking for yourself. This process will give you the time to examine information, build discernment, and make the decisions that shape your destiny.

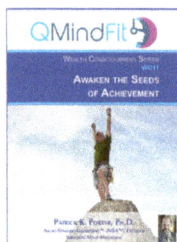

WC11 – Awaken the Seeds of Achievement

Now you can arouse the sleeping seeds of greatness that will carry you to heights you might never have dreamed possible. The key to this process is controlled attention. By learning to fix your attention on what you want, instead of what you don't want, prosperity and harmony will be the natural byproduct.

WC12 – Harness the Power of
Cooperative Effort

During this visualization, you will move beyond mastermind groups into a coordinated effort to work with a team spirit that includes definiteness of purpose and absolute harmony.

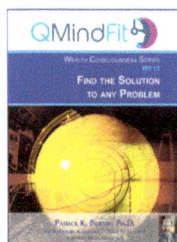

WC13 – Find the Solution to Any Problem

Albert Einstein was fond of saying, "You can never solve a problem on the level at which it was created." What Einstein understood is the power within the other-than-conscious mind to dwell on solutions instead of problems. Soon you will see problems for what they really are—temporary setbacks and stepping stones to success.

WC14 – Tap Into The Creative
Vision of Infinite Intelligence

Wealth streams to those who work smarter not harder. In this creative visualization you will make the inner connection with the guiding force that lets you accomplish the impossible. Through this inner faith the path to wealth is illuminated.

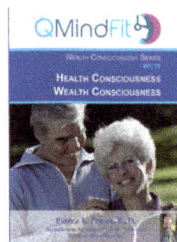

WC15 – Health Consciousness, Wealth Consciousness

There is a universal truth that what the mind dreams about the body brings about. Balance in mind and body is key to wealth consciousness. In this process, you will plan a life of wealth, health, and abundance from the inside out.

WC16 – Employ the Power of Time For Wealth Consciousness

In this program you will discover how the captains of industry used assertiveness and diplomacy to get what they want. You will keep the dream stealers and time bandits out of your life so you can keep your eye on the prize and enjoy the ride to riches.

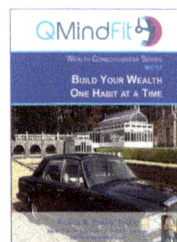

WC17 – Build Your Wealth One Habit at a Time

Just as nature adheres to strict laws, the person of wealth lives by the laws of excellence. Making positive choices becomes a driving power in your life as you master the power of thought. Your other-then-conscious mind will become your guide in building unlimited wealth.

Habits of Naturally Thin People
Patrick K. Porter, Ph.D.

Have you ever looked at a naturally thin person and wondered how they seem to look at food in such a different way than you do? How some people can leave junk foods and unhealthy foods alone and crave healthy, vibrant, alive foods? It is possible to change your unhealthy behaviors and create new, healthy habits that will serve you for a lifetime. In this audio series, Dr. Patrick Porter (PhD) will help you discover how, by using the Q MindFit you will learn healthier habits to help you create the life you want to live. You can learn how to conquer cravings, increase your self-confidence and learn the habits of naturally thin individuals. Each week you will take another step toward a lifetime of healthy living and supercharge your motivation with these powerful Q MindFit audio sessions! You will eliminate the problem where it started--in your own mind. With Q MindFit you can change your habits and develop healthy new ones!

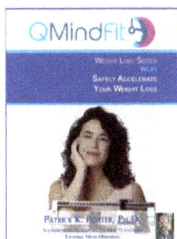

WL01 – Safely Speeding Up Weight Loss

In this powerful audio session, you'll learn the habits necessary to help you think, act and respond like a naturally thin person. Your sense of worth will improve when you discover and use inner resources you never even knew you had. Sit back, relax, and learn how to develop the healthy habits necessary to turn your body into a fat-burning machine—and learn the behaviors that can help you to keep the weight off forever!

WL02 – Simple Steps for Self-Confidence for Weight Control

When you learn these simple steps for self-confidence, you will unleash your creative mind, allowing your mind and body to work together for lasting weight loss. Dr. Patrick Porter will help you envision your own bright and compelling future—a future where all your physical, mental and emotional goals have been reached. You'll awaken with complete confidence in your new, healthy behaviors, aware that your future is filled with infinite possibilities!

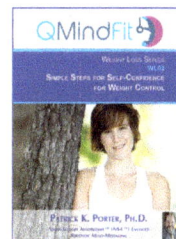

WL03 – Eliminate the Gain/Loss Cycle

End the yo-yo dieting cycle! With this motivational SMT process, you'll let go of the past, because the past no longer controls you. The present is your most powerful moment, and in the present you're free to make the choices that can help you realize and maintain your natural and ideal weight forever.

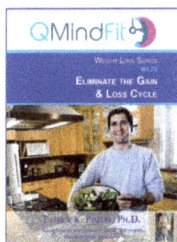

WL04 – Producing Success One Thought at a Time

Every day, thoughts move through your mind, many without your awareness. In this session, Dr. Patrick Porter helps you learn to overcome the negative thoughts, patterns and beliefs that have been keeping you from reaching your goals. As you release the negative thoughts, you'll free yourself to enjoy more joy and success than you ever thought possible!

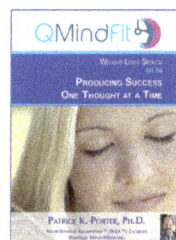

WL05 – Sunrise Agreement

As you experience this dynamic audio session by Dr. Patrick Porter, your old habits and new desires will communicate and create a contract for success. With this "Sunrise Agreement," you'll awaken knowing every day is a new day, a gift that you can use to create the changes you desire. Most of all, you'll experience every day with the power to use your mind and body to improve your life at the most powerful moment possible—now!

WL06 – Create Your Weight Loss Support Team

Having the proper support is important to maintaining the healthy new behaviors you're learning. With this audio session, you will learn to build a caring and supportive team that will improve every relationship. With this type of attitude you will create all the support you need to reach your goals.

WL07 – Developing Positive Eating Patterns

Deep inside, your body knows what it needs to operate at its full, vibrant potential. With this session, you'll mentally journey back to a time when you enjoyed doing the best for your body. When you bring those skills back with you to the present, you'll find yourself more comfortable and confident each day, effortlessly eating the right foods at the right times. Above all, you'll know that appetite is of the mind, but hunger is of the body!

WL08 – Turn Up Your Fat-Burning Thermostat

Use self-mastery technology to rehearse habits and behaviors that will help you create a healthy new life. These simple tips are the keys to learning what you need to do to create the life you've always imagined.

WL09 – Motivation for Monday Morning

In the past, Monday mornings have always seemed the ideal time to start changes in your life. The problem came when that Monday morning motivation faded throughout the week. With this inspiring process by Dr. Patrick Porter, you'll learn to recapture that beginning-of-the-week motivation and use it every day of the week. One day at a time, you'll know that every day, in every way, you're getting better and better at making the changes you desire.

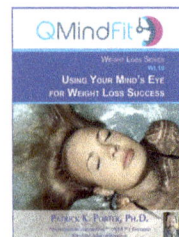

WL10 – Using Your Mind's Eye for Weight-Loss Success

Enter the theater of your mind and watch your own weight-loss success take place before your eyes. Success will follow you as naturally as your shadow when you solve the problems of your past with solutions you see in your present and future. Most of all, you'll awaken a feeling of success in you today, knowing that the accomplishments you see in your mind's eye will happen in your body naturally, one day at a time.

WL11 – Stop Dieting and Start Living

Your mind has a natural ability for removing the mental obstacles that are keeping you from realizing your goals. You will discover why appetite is of the mind and hunger is of the body. You can plan a lifetime of healthy habits, thoughts and actions.

WL12 – Exercising is Energizing

Wouldn't you love to have fun exercising? With this process by Dr. Patrick Porter, you'll develop the habits and behaviors of a person who naturally loves to exercise. You'll use your creative mind to imagine, and then do, physical activities you enjoy. When you're in complete, optimistic control of your mind and body, you'll see excellence in the naturally-thin people around you and develop the same abilities in your own life.

WL13 – Take Back Control of Your Appetite

The average person gains up to four pounds a year. That's a 40-pound weight gain in ten short years! This audio session was developed to help you learn new behaviors to break that cycle. You will be visualizing success by seeing yourself overcoming poor eating habits and the guilt feelings often associated with those poor eating habits. You will discover why true happiness starts when you eat to live… And eliminate any thought of living to eat!

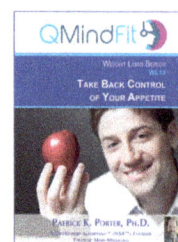

Patrick K. Porter, Ph.D. - Audio Session Catalog

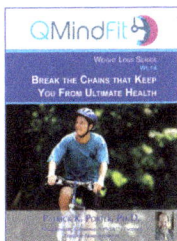

WL14 – Break the Chains that Keep You from Ultimate Health

Break the bonds of the past that keep you tied to foods and habits that no longer serve you. With this process, you'll find it easy to create a new reality where you are no longer imprisoned by negative thoughts, patterns or beliefs. Instead, Dr. Patrick Porter will help you open the treasure chest of your natural talents, skills and abilities, and awaken yourself to the freedom of today.

WL15 – Stay Fit Through Healthy Eating Patterns

Your body image starts in your mind. Using powerful motivation you can unlock the unlimited potential within you! With this audio session you can learn to change the habits that caused you to gain weight and then choose the habits and behaviors you need to remain naturally thin for life. You can stay on track when you forget about dieting and make simple lifestyle changes.

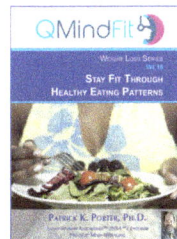

WL16 – Extinguish Junk Food Cravings

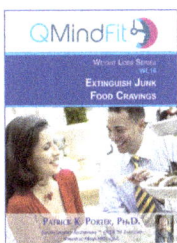

Let this SMT audio session help you learn new behaviors to leave the junk food habit in the past. You'll visualize steps you can take to end binge eating and transform your appetite so you'll crave the healthy foods that are more in line with your present goals. Imagine your joy when you feel confident at every meal. Using the power of your mind, you can learn to leave your unhealthy eating patterns in the past.

WL17 – Quick Tips To Lose Weight Even If You Eat Out Every day

Eating out can be a treat and a timesaver. Someone else does the cooking and there are no dishes to do. Now you can extend that joy by making healthy choices—even if your choice isn't on the menu. You will discover how to take back control of your health by taking control of your food choices. There's no reason you can't enjoy eating out with family and friends and still have a naturally thin body. We'll help you learn how to plan for success no matter what the circumstances!

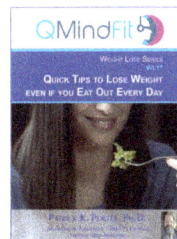

WL18 – Eliminate The Traps Associated With Dieting

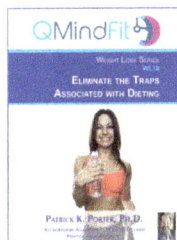

Dieting traps can vary from Monday morning blues to Friday night fever—traps almost every dieter has fallen prey to. Now discover how to avoid these dieting traps by using your creative mind to rehearse all your best intentions. Soon you will find yourself demonstrating the habits and behaviors of a naturally thin person no matter the weather, your mood, or the day of the week. When you choose to become a conscious creator in your weight loss journey, success becomes as natural as breathing.

WL19 – Visualize & Realize a Lifetime of Weight Loss Success

No one wants to have to diet over and over again. This session will reframe the old patterns and behaviors that held you back in the past so you feel free to lose weight once and for all. You will make peace with your past, realizing that the past was a proving ground for the future. As you master the art of relaxation, you will instead visualize a lifetime of new behaviors that can be realized in a very effective, easy and fun way!

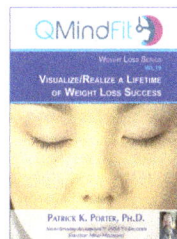

WL20 – Making the Connection for Permanent Weight Loss

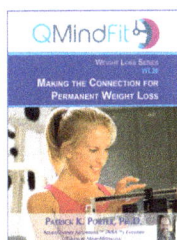

You will use your mind to discover the secrets of naturally thin people and learn how to implement them in your life to get the results you want. Once you know the truth, the dieting lie that chained you to overweight habits will melt away. With this connection, true health will be yours and negative thoughts about yourself will never again control you.

Habits of Naturally Thin People

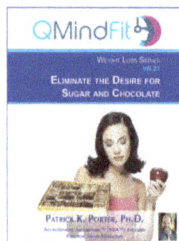

WL21 – Eliminate the Desire for Sugar & Chocolate

When you use your mind's natural abilities, eliminating your cravings for sweet, starchy and even fatty foods is possible. You will learn to focus on creating the cravings for positive, life-giving foods that are fresh and alive. From this new mindset, you'll respond to foods with health in mind. You will explore the possibility that nothing taste as good as thin feels!

WL22 – Self Control And Radiant Health

When you learn to erase all doubt from your mind, you can stay purposeful and on track with your health goals. Can you imagine how wonderful it will feel to display discipline and confidence when it's enjoyable and fun? Well, that's exactly what Dr. Patrick Porter has done for you in this life-affirming session.

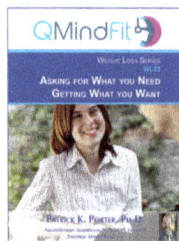

WL23 – Asking For What You Need and Getting What You Want

Do you know how to say no to people? Do you know how to ask for what your want? If you've had trouble communicating your needs and wants in the past, this audio session will help you to achieve success using these exciting new communication skills. You will visualize yourself communicating with others with assertiveness and confidence. You will learn to create powerful, fulfilling relationships. You will get more out of life and have fun in the process.

WL24 – Choosing Habits That Keep You Naturally-Thin

Unleash the power of selective thinking and learn to choose the foods and activities that are healthiest for your body. Eliminate the need for the dead, devitalized foods of the past as you remember . . . "Its not for me, but for my body, that I eat healthy foods." You will build a lifestyle that will support you in staying naturally thin.

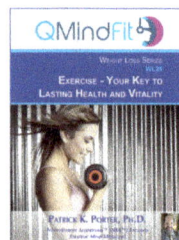

WL25 – Exercise - Your Key To Lasting Health & Vitality

With this visualization you will create enthusiasm for health and exercise. You will mentally rehearse an active new lifestyle where exercise is fun and enjoyable. Imagine how good you will feel as you burn fat, build muscle, and sculpt the body you want. Warning...listening to this audio session may transform your body into a fat burning machine!

WL26 – Breezing Through the Weekends Naturally Thin

Many diets start on Monday and end before Thursday. Learning to maintain your desired goals through the weekend may seem like a tall order. But, now you can get off the weekly weight loss roller coaster. This audio session is specially designed to help you keep your goals in high gear even on the weekend. Imagine the joy of starting the week with unlimited confidence!

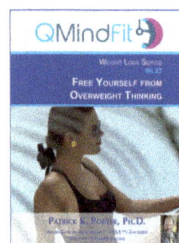

WL27– Free Yourself from Overweight Thinking

As you develop the habits associated with naturally thin individuals, it's important to unlock the gates of your mind and release the past. Once you develop healthy new habits and behaviors, you free yourself from fat-induced discomfort. Dr. Patrick Porter will help you build your new body image; you'll envision the future where you are healthy, confident, slim and attractive.

WL28 – Make Exercise An Automatic Part Of Your Life

People who learn to enjoy exercise find that this healthy habit helps them maintain their weight loss goals. In this SMT session you will find powerful motivation to exercise, which is your key to lasting energy. When exercise is automatic and fun, you create a more active lifestyle.

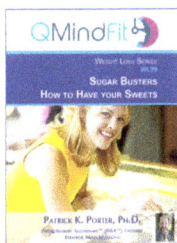

WL29 – Sugar Busters … How to Have Your Sweets and Lose Weight, Too

Even naturally thin people eat sweets from time to time. Now you can, too—without guilt or shame. In this SMT session Dr. Patrick Porter will show you how you can occasionally eat sweets without derailing your weight loss goals. Enjoying these foods occasionally doesn't have to burden you with guilt. Your new healthy habits will keep your goals in sight.

WL30 – Learn the 10 to 1 Method for Giving Your Body What It Needs

In this process you will start to learn to master SMT on your own. Imagine learning new habits and behaviors that help you throughout the day to think and eat like a naturally thin person. That is exactly what Dr. Patrick Porter guides you to do with this deeply relaxing visualization.

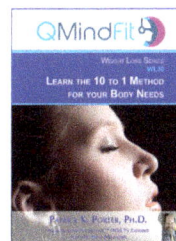

WL31 – Make Your Daily Activities Your Daily Motivation

During this audio session you will close your eyes, sit back, relax, and rehearse how your daily routines can turn into excitement as you mentally cleanse your mind and body and discover the true you. By knowing what you want and learning to follow through—even when you don't want to—you build the habits of a naturally thin person.

WL32 – Make Your Motivation to Exercise Sizzle!

Exercise is fun when you feel motivated. Now you can get that edge with these creative tools that build your motivation and drive. While listening to this audio session you'll learn how to develop an effective and lasting exercise program. You'll be turning fat into lean body mass by using your mind to make exercise fun.

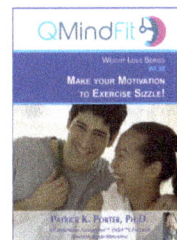

WL33 – Building Your Self-confidence and Self-esteem

If you've ever failed at dieting, you've lived the frustration and disappointment that follows. In this session Dr. Porter will help you leave behind all that negativity for good. You'll then discover fun and creative ways to accentuate the positive and transform your thoughts, actions and beliefs into those of a healthy, happy slim person.

WL34 – Unlocking Your Innate Intelligence to Re-create Your Body

Get ready to unlock the power of choice as you use your body's innate intelligence to stop the war within you. In this process, Dr. Porter will show you the difference between power and force. When you make peace with your body, you don't have to force it to do anything. You'll then find it possible to make changes in your habits that reflect those of naturally thin people.

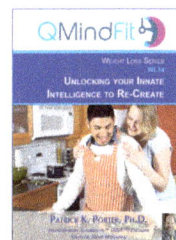

WL35 – Using Assertiveness in Weight Control

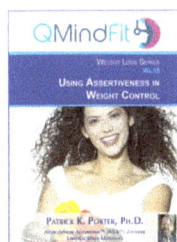

It's easy to say yes or no when you are steadfastly focused on your health goals. Dr. Porter will help you experience progressive relaxation while you plan your life as a naturally thin person. Understanding the hidden secrets behind the power words of yes and no will set you free from the emotional roller coaster of the lose/gain cycle. Rehearsing when and where to use these power words will help you achieve your weight loss and health goals for life.

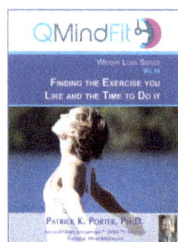

WL36 – Finding the Exercise You Like and the Time to Do It

Without proper motivation, some people choose destructive or limiting behaviors that may sabotage their weight loss goals. During this audio session, Dr. Patrick Porter will help you create a healthy environment where exercise fits into your busy lifestyle. Learn to create balance in your home and work life so you can develop the habits and behaviors of a thin person.

WL37 – Accept and Love Your Body

We tend to give the most attention to those we care about most. Now is the time to give your body the loving care it needs and deserves. When you learn to build a positive relationship with yourself by loving and accepting your body, you can learn to make better choices that fit in with your new goals. Plus, all of your relationships will improve. It all starts with your thoughts.

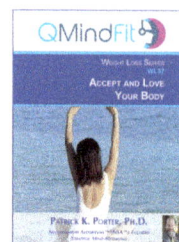

WL38 – Gain Power Over Your Appetite

During this session, Dr. Porter will help you discover how appetite is of the mind and true hunger is of the body. You will learn to recognize the difference between appetite and hunger so you can make food choices from a place of self-empowerment. You can develop the behavior of eating only when you are truly hungry and automatically stopping when you are full. You'll experience the truth--that power stems from choice, and you will choose to eat only what your body needs.

WL39 – Staying on Track with Your Transition to Thinness

Everyday you are bombarded with over 50,000 messages, each one prompting you to think or act in certain ways - no wonder staying focused can seem impossible! Dr. Porter will help you to get and stay focused on what's most important to you—your transition to a healthier, happier lifestyle.

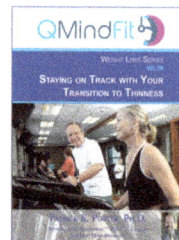

WL40 – Eliminate Your Weight Loss Enemies For Good

During this audio session, Dr. Porter will teach you to eliminate those old enemies that kept you trapped in the negative programming of the past. Whether it's food, family, friends, or your own self-talk, you will relax and allow your other-than-conscious mind to work out success on your terms.

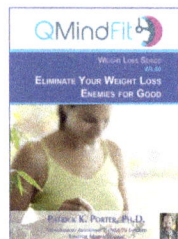

WL41 – Plan a Healthy Home and Workplace

Now you can build the skills necessary for creating balance in your home, work, and personal life. These are the skills that will have you learning the habits of naturally thin people. During this audio session, Dr. Patrick Porter will teach you ways to motivate yourself, to learn the habits that naturally thin people possess, and to leave in the past any destructive or limiting behaviors that may otherwise sabotage your weight loss goals.

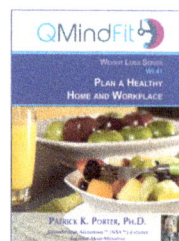

WL42 – Supercharge Your Self-image

Your self-image is the way you think about yourself; and it directly affects the food choices you make. With this SMT program, you will learn powerful new habits and behaviors to empower you to enjoy fresh and alive foods as much or more than the old junk foods of the past. You will learn to savor the flavors in fresh, natural foods. You will also learn to take pleasure in the energy that you derive from the foods that promote lasting weight-loss results. And along the way you will be building a healthy image of yourself.

WL43 – Eliminate Fear And Stay Naturally Thin

Dr. Porter will help you to overcome fear-of-failure thinking, the primary factor in disappointing weight-loss results. Allow this powerful SMT audio session to help you develop a mindset of success. When you eliminate fear-of-failure thinking, there's nothing stopping you from reaching your goals.

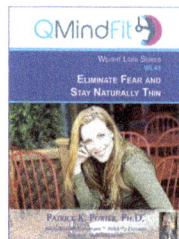

WL44 – Mental Toughness for Weight Management

During this SMT program, you will create a rock-solid positive attitude about being naturally thin and staying at your natural and ideal weight. This process mentally trains you to generate resources where and when you need them to accomplish your health goals. With so many forces seeming to work against you, you will come to realize that your needs are just as important as everyone else's.

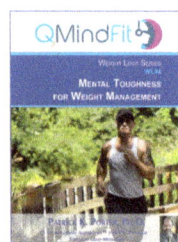

Patrick K. Porter, Ph.D. - Audio Session Catalog

WL45 – Increasing Self-Esteem and Optimism

Self-esteem is an inside job. In this session, you will learn to calm and steady your emotions by allowing yourself to relax with this audio session. You will create the habit of optimism, leaving behind fear, frustration, and anxiety while journeying on a peaceful mental vacation. With this overall feeling of wellbeing, you can learn the habits and behaviors necessary to accomplish your health and weight goals.

WL46 – Conquering Cravings for Sugar and Unhealthy Fats

Use this powerful audio session to help you leave those old enemies that kept you trapped in the lose/gain cycle in your past. Whether your cravings are related to stress, hormones, habit, or your own self-talk, relax and allow your other-than-conscious mind to work out success on your terms.

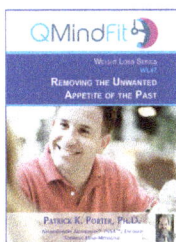

WL47 – Removing the Unwanted Appetite of the Past

Now you can harness the power of your mind to overcome any past programming. At the same time, you will learn to recognize true hunger, which is a different feeling from appetite. You will learn how to unlock the power of possibility thinking and feel the habits of a naturally thin person grow within you.

WL48 – Healthy Eating During the Holidays

Recapture the joy of the holidays. Why suffer or feel deprived when everyone else is having a good time? When you focus your mind on the positive experiences, and develop the habits of a naturally thin person, your holidays will be a delightful experience once again.

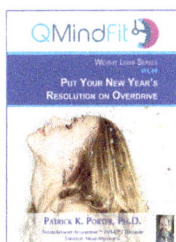

WL49 – Put Your New Year's Resolutions on Overdrive

Tap into the limitless motivation of your mind to stay on track, build unstoppable resolve, and accomplish your resolutions. You can learn the habits of naturally thin people as your confidence builds and your life improves!

WL50 – Giving Thanks and Staying Slim

Many people find themselves gaining weight over the holiday season. Allow this SMT audio session to help you create healthy holidays. This audio session will take you step-by-step through the Thanksgiving season, helping you leave behind the poor eating habits and the guilt and stress associated with those habits. Eat less and enjoy the holidays more – you can't beat that combination!

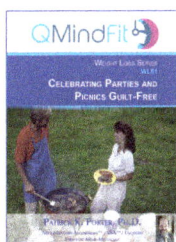

WL51 – Celebrating Parties and Picnics Guilt-Free

Are you too worried about your eating habits to enjoy parties and picnics? Can't enjoy yourself while everyone else is having fun? With this audio session you'll learn the habit of enjoying good times with friends and family without the worry, deprivation, or guilt of the past.

WL52 – Keeping It Off with a Naturally Thin Mindset

Imagine your life after you find fun ways of focusing on yourself at your natural and healthy weight. Dr. Patrick Porter will help you discover how, by developing an awareness of who you truly are, you can learn and maintain the habits and behaviors of a naturally thin person. You will keep your focus on health, and your weight will take care of itself.

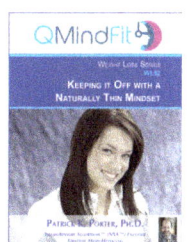

If you are the proud owner of one of these:

CLARITY

CALM

COPING

=

CONFIDENCE

You need the nutrition that EMPowerPlus™ Q96 provides.

— Tony Stephan

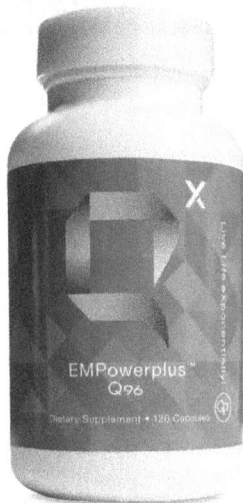

Did you know your brain weighs only 2 to 4 pounds of your total body weight but utilizes up to 50% of the nutrients your body consumes? Make sure you provide your brain the nutrition it needs with **EMPowerplus™ Q96**.*

Backed by years of scientific research, **EMPowerplus™ Q96** is specifically formulated to provide essential nutritional support to the brain. **EMPowerplus™ Q96** delivers a balanced blend of 36 vitamins, minerals and amino acids in a safe and effective dose to support mood stability, mental clarity, improved cognition, and overall brain health and function for both children and adults.*

EMPowerplus™ Q96 is one of the **most-researched micronutrient formula** in the world with 25 independent clinical trials and medical studies and is unlike any other vitamin or mineral supplement on the market.*

*These statements have not been evaluated by the food and drug administration. This product is not intended to diagnose, treat, cure or prevent any disease.

Live Life eXponentially!

EMPowerplus™ Q96
Dietary Supplement • 120 Capsules

Supplement Facts

Serving Size: 4 Capsules
Servings Per Container: 30

Amount Per Serving		% Daily Value
Vitamin A (as retinyl palmitate)	1536 IU	30%
Vitamin C (as ascorbic acid)	160 mg	267%
Vitamin D (as cholecalciferol)	384 IU	100%
Vitamin E (as d-alpha tocopheryl acid succinate)	100IU	320%
Thiamine (as thiamine mononitrate)	4.8 mg	320%
Riboflavin	3.6 mg	210%
Niacin (as niacinamide)	24 mg	120%
Vitamin B6 (as pyridoxine hydrochloride)	9.6 mg	480%
Folic Acid	384 mcg	100%
Vitamin B12 (as cyanocobalamin)	240 mcg	4000%
Biotin	288 mcg	100%
Pantothenic Acid (as d-calcium pantothenate)	5.8 mg	60%
Iron (as chelate)	3.7 mg	20%
Iodine (from Atlantic kelp)	54.4 mcg	36%

Q Sciences Proprietary Nano Blend 2,249 mg
Calcium chelate, Magnesium chelate, Potassium chelate, Phosphorus chelate, Copper chelate, Zinc chelate, Manganese chelate, Selenium chelate, Molybdenum chelate

Q Sciences Proprietary Optimization Blend 670 mg
Choline bitartrate, DL-phenylalanine, Citrus bioflavonoids, Inositol, L-glutamine, L-methionine, Grape seed extract, Ginkgo biloba leaf, Germanium sesquioxide, Boron chelate, Vanadium chelate, Nickel chelate

Other Ingredients: Capsule Shell (Gelatin, Titanium dioxide), Microcrystalline cellose, Glycine, Magnesium stearate, Citric acid, Silicon dioxide, Mineral wax

Live Life eXponentially!

Q

Cellerciser

The Cellerciser is an innovative piece of fitness equipment designed to take your fat burning workouts and strengthening exercises to the next level. By flexing 75 trillion cells in the body nearly 100 times a minute, this home-exercise rebounder enhances fitness by combining isometric, isotonic, callisthenic, aerobic, and flexibility workouts into just one daily 10-minute session.*

Why the Cellerciser?

There are many forms of exercise and most work the body as individual muscles or muscle groups. Since there are so many areas of the body to target, typical exercise programs can take up a lot of time and require costly exercise equipment. The Cellerciser gives you that full-body workout in the privacy of your own home in a more efficient and cost-effective manner.*

Features:

- Triple-tiered carbon steel anodized springs
- Safe and durable with all-steel construction
- Perfect for in-home use
- Safe for people of all ages and fitness levels*
- Efficient workout in just 10 minutes a day*

KEY BENEFITS:

- Reduces stress*
- Burns calories*
- Stimulates lymphatic system *
- Builds and tones muscle*
- Strengthens heart and cellular efficiency*

Live Life eXponentially!

What the media has to say about Self-Mastery Technology . . .

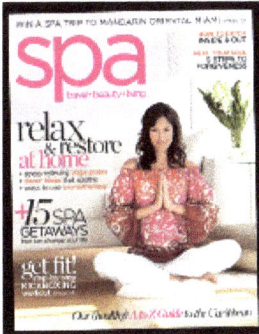

Health Report—Creative Visualization

Want to drop pounds, quit smoking, or stress less? Then consider guided visualization. A technique used by psychologists since the late 1800s, it is now being offered at spas, too—such as Mezzanine Spa in New York City and The TreeHouse in Venice Beach, California – through a program called Creative Visualization and Relaxation (CVR). The brainchild of Dr. Patrick Porter, CVR utilizes flashing LEDs and sound pulses to guide you into a relaxed state bordering on sleep in which suggestions reach deeper than they can when the mind is alert. During each of the more than 300 CVR programs available, you are asked to visualize yourself in various scenarios to train your mind to react to old triggers with new behaviors. There's also a personal version that lets you take the power of positive thinking with you wherever you go.

By: Anne-Marie Cook
Spa Magazine

o o o

Envision Yourself to Better Health

Guided imagery is similar to meditation, except that the focus of your thought is a physical part of the body you'd like to strengthen. The process of picturing a healthy heart or a svelte body can lower stress levels and help you "see" what it would feel like to be well.

High-tech Guided Imagery

You don't necessarily have to shell out big bucks for a personalized coach to reap the benefits of guided imagery . . . self-administered mental coaching programs can help you conquer bad habits or initiate good habits just by envisioning it— sitting back in your favorite easy chair, taking a deep breath, and completely relaxing every muscle in the body. A critical element . . . is light and sound technology to make your brain more receptive to the coaching. Just as the stimuli of music beats and flashing lights at a night club affect your brain . . . light and sound technology bring your brain frequency to a state called theta. The theta state is a meditative one that reportedly leads to higher levels of creativity, learning and inspiration.

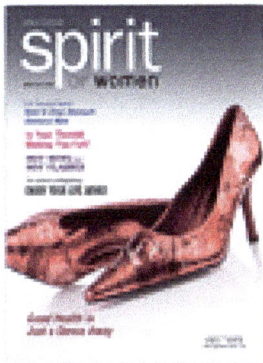

By: *Spirit of Women*
Spring 2008

The "Wellness Revolution" is Sweeping the Nation

Forward thinking hospitals that address patient demand for total wellness are now providing creative visualization and relaxation (CVR) mental coaching for their patients.

o o o

By: *Lenny LaCour*
PULSE Magazine

The Once-a-day Stress Relief Formula
"FOR ME AND ONLY ME"

Science proves that if you don't process your day-to-day experiences, they stay in your sub-conscious and keep you awake. Relaxation and exercise, yoga, music and the overall environment can help. It's getting back to the basics of the mind, body and spirit.

Self-Mastery Technology

Dr. Patrick Porter explained that it's important to take a few minutes during the day to just unplug your phone and become consciously aware of your thoughts. If you slow down mentally, you become more aware of your unconscious thinking. Basically, we clog up our minds to the point where we can't focus on positive thoughts. Porter's theory is that our mind works in blocks of information. The conscious mind can only store several chunks at a time, and the rest of the thoughts remain in the subconscious waiting to be resolved. It's important to clear your mind to allow the wind to blow the thoughts through.

Dr. Porter's program is based on creative visualization and relaxation (CVR). Sessions result in stress release, clearer thinking, improved memory and enhanced creativity—a spiritual journey within yourself indeed.

o   o   o

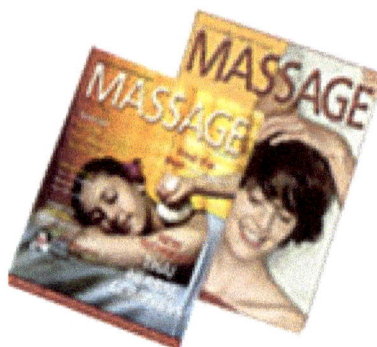

The New Generation of Mind-Body Therapies—Biofeedback and Brain Training

Massage therapist Leslie White uses the biofeedin equipment and Dr. Patrick Porter's soothing voice to full advantage during her massage sessions. She said the combination of light, pulsating sound and "Dr. Porter's very pleasant voice softly saying, 'Now you will feel her hands massaging,'" really helps the clients "focus on themselves."

o   o   o

By: Chris Cunningham
Massage Magazine

By: *Kelly Hushin*
BeautyNewsNYC.com

Meditation at the Mezzanine Spa

"After about 15 minutes, it was as though my mind and body were at one. It was similar to the feeling you get when you're almost asleep and then have a sort of "mini-dream" that brings you back to the waking world."

o   o   o

Researchers tested novice meditators on a button-pressing task requiring speed and concentration. Performance was greater after 40 minutes of meditation than after a 40-minute nap.

The Boston Globe
November 23, 2005

What the research has to say about
Frequency Following Response. . .

Dr. Roger K. Cady, Dr. Norman Shealy in "Neurochemical Responses to Cranial Electrical Stimulation and Photo-Stimulation via Brain Wave Synchronization."Study performed by the Shealy Institute of Comprehensive Health Care, Springfield, Missouri, 1990, 11 pp.:

Eleven patients had peridural and blood analysis performed before and after the relaxation sessions using flash emitting goggles. An average increase of beta-endorphin levels of 25% and serotonin levels of 21% were registered. The beta-endorphin levels are comparative to those obtained by cranial electrical stimulation (CES). This indicates a potential decrease of depression related symptoms when using photic stimulation.

o   o   o

Dr. Norman Shealy, Dr. Richard Cox In `Pain Reduction and Relaxation with Brain Wave Synchronization (Photo-Stimulation). Study performed by the Forest Institute of Professional Psychology, Springfield, Missouri, 1990, 9pp.

Cerebral synchronization was obtained with photic stimulation devices and tested on more than 5,000 patients suffering from chronic pain and stress-symptoms during the `80s. A detailed study on 92 patients indicated that 88 obtained relaxation results higher than 60% after 30- minute sessions at 10 hz. Thirty patients had sessions in Theta (5 hz) and experienced relaxation states of 50–100% after five minutes as well as improved pain relief. Eight patients had blood tests before and after the sessions and showed improved beta-endorphin levels of 10–50%. All of these relaxation results are improved when combining the photic stimulation with relaxation audio tapes.

o   o   o

Dr. Thomas Budzynski in "Biofeedback and the Twilight States of Consciousness," in G.E. Schwartz and D. Shapiro eds., Consciousness and Self-Regulation, vol. 1, New York, Plenum 1976 and non-published studies at the Biofeedback Institute of Denver, 1980:

Using a first-generation prototype, Dr. Budzynski concluded that "these devices produce a distinct relaxation state. Programming the device between 3 and 7 hz, it takes about 10 to 15 minutes for the patients to enter--effortlessly-a state of hypnosis. They terminate the sessions relaxed and with a feeling of well-being." Also, "the device has a calming effect on nervous or anxious patients. In a majority of cases the patients feel relaxed and calm during a period of three to four days after the session. It happens that the subjects have a reminiscence of childhood experiences, particularly when in Theta. They related their experiences which we incorporated into our psychotherapeutic program."

o   o   o

Dr. Gene W. Brockopp, Review of Research on Multi-Modal Sensory Stimulation with Clinical Implications and Research Proposals (non-published,1984):

Dr. Brockopp analyzed audio-visual brain stimulation and in particular hemispheric synchronization during EEG monitoring. "By inducing hemispheric coherence the machine can contribute to improved intellectual functioning of the brain. Like children spending most of their time in Theta, the machine allows a reduction in learning time. With adults a return into Theta allows them to rediscover childhood experiences. The machine is like a `lost and found office' for the subconscious."

Dr. Brockopp's conclusion is that dissipative structures allow the mind-via audio-visual stimulation-to abandon certain present neurological structures in order to maintain a higher, more coherent and flexible state of consciousness, thus allowing for improved communication of neuro-entities.

o   o   o

Dr. Norman Thomas and David Siever, University of Alberta, Florida. Several publications, notably: The Effect of Repetitive Audio/Visual Stimulation in Skeletomotor and Vasomotor Activity, 1989:

"We stimulated one of two groups of 30 people with a brain-stimulation device to test relaxation levels, using 10 hz frequency while observing their muscular tension with an EMG and their index skin temperature. The second group had to relax without machines via traditional means of autosuggestion. Most of the people in the second group said they felt relaxed while demonstrating greater tension (EMG) and lower skin temperatures, both of which are stress and nervous tension indicators. The group using the machine obtained deep relaxation state going beyond the programmed 15 minutes. EMG curves confirmed relaxation of the cortex due to the frequency adoption response."

These findings were also verified by James Greene and Dr. E.J. Baukus of FOCUS Human Research Development in Bourdonnais, Illinois. The muscular tension curve of the trapezius muscle were indicative of deep muscular relaxation.

o o o

Dr. Robert Cosgrove, Jr. of the anesthesia department of Stanford University School of Medicine, Stanford, California.

Dr. Cosgrove proceeded in 1988 with multiple experiences with the same devices and concluded that states of deep relaxation are obtained with these machines. "We are very optimistic about the possibilities of calming our patients before and after surgery. By the way, we already treat chronic stress affected patients. Thus, our EEG analysis shows that optimal cerebral functioning can be obtained with regular use of such audio-visual apparatus. The machines could eventually slow the decreasing cerebral performance with the elderly. This type of machine could 'revolutionize neurology and medicine.'"

o o o

Dale S. Foster of Memphis State University, "EEG and Subjective Correlates of Alpha Frequency Binaural Beats Stimulation Combined with Alpha Biofeedback," 1988:

Mr. Foster's conclusions indicate that the combination of binaural sounds with audio-visual stimulation machines allow access into Alpha states of consciousness much faster than with traditional biofeedback techniques.

Elisabeth Philipos, Pepperdine University, California, and James McGaugh, University of California, Irvine, have tested the effects of Theta frequencies on learning.

During their study a group of 20 students learned 1,800 words of Bulgarian in 120 hours while using Theta stimulation programs. In about 1/3 of normal time they spoke and wrote the new language.

D.J. Anderson, B.Sc., M.B., "The Treatment of Migraine with Variable Frequency Photo-Stimulation," in Headache, March 1989, pp 154–155:
D.J. Anderson used photo-stimulating goggles with variable frequency using red LEDs in order to stimulate the optic nerve, through closed eyes, right and left with frequencies between 0.5 and 50 hz. The study included seven patients who suffered a total of more than 50 migraines during the observation period. Forty-nine of these migraines were relieved (either by reducing the average duration or by increasing the frequency interval in between migraine crisis) and 36 other migraines could be stopped while using the goggles.

o o o

Dr. Glen D. Solomon, "Slow Wave Photic Stimulation in the Treatment of Headache-A Preliminary Report," in Headache, November 1985, pp 444–447:
Dr. Solomon works for the Department of Internal Medicine at the U.S. Air Force Medical Center in Scott, Illinois, where 24 patients with chronic headaches and migraines were treated with photic stimulation apparatus at 5–8 hz frequency. Fourteen of 15 patients with sustained headaches and 5 of 6 patients with chronic headaches noticed complete relief after the treatment. Four patients treated with the same photo-stimulation apparatus showed no reaction.

o o o

Bruce Harrah-Confort, Ph.D., Indiana University, "Alpha and Theta Response to the MindsEye Plus," 1990:
The study included 15 persons between the ages of 24 and 38 years old who were asked to relax via auto-suggestion with headphones dispensing a synthetic sound (100 cycles at 60 hz) and then to use the audio-visual stimulator MindsEye Plus™. EEG graphic analysis showed that the first relaxation method did not alter the EEG-trace significantly vs. normal. MindsEye Plus users had, however, strongly improved Alpha and Theta tracings and experienced profound relaxation. There were also signs that would validate hemispheric synchronization during the experience.

o o o

Joseph Glickson, Department of Psychology, Tel Aviv University, "Photic Driving and Altered States of Consciousness: An Exploratory Study," in Imagination, Cognition and Personality, vol. 6(2), 1986–87, pp 167–182:
Four persons were exposed to photic stimulation in the 18, 10 and 6 hz ranges. A frequency response was established by two subjects during the initial session according to EEG measurements. These persons had an altered state of consciousness, and reported their visual and auditive experiences. The two other subjects had similar experiences during follow-on sessions. The study concludes that photic entrainment provokes altered states of consciousness according to the applied frequencies.

o o o

Paul Williams and Michael West, Department of Psychological Medicine, University Hospital of Wales and University of Wales Institute of Science and Technology, Cardiff, Wales, "EEG Responses to Photic Stimulation in Persons Experienced in Meditation," in Electroencephalography and Clinical Neurophysiology, 1975, 39, pp 519-522:
Williams and West tested photic entrainment on two test groups of 10 people. The test group produced significantly more Alpha waves and smaller Alpha blocking compared to the control group familiar with traditional meditation techniques. Alpha induction was realized faster and more frequently within the test vs. the control group.

Tsuyoshi Inouye, Noboru Sumitsuji and Kazuo Matsumoto, Department of Neuropsychiatry, Osaka University Medical School, Japan, "EEG Changes Induced by Light Stimuli Modulated with the Subject's Alpha Rhythm," in Electroencephalography and Clinical Neurophysiology, 1980, 49, pp 135–142:
Seven of nine persons undergoing the test obtained occipital Alpha of both hemispheres and concurrently coherence and phase between right and left occipital EEG. These results tend to confirm a hemispheric synchronization tendency by subjects using photic stimulation in the 10 hz (Alpha frequency) range.

o o o

Ronald Lesser, Hans Luders, G. Klem and Dudley Dinner, Department of Neurology, Cleveland Clinic Foundation, "Visual Potentials Evoked by Light- Emitting Diodes Mounted in Goggles," in Cleveland Clinic Quarterly, vol. 52, No. 2, Summer 1985, pp. 223–228:
A comparison of stimulation by strobiscopic lights and LED diodes shows that both methods have similar effects. LED stimulation may be preferable in intensive care units or during surgery because the type of stimulus is less disturbing.

o o o

Richard E. Townsend, Ph.D. of Neuropsychiatric Research, U.S. Naval Hospital in San Diego, "A Device for Generation and Presentation of Modulated Light Stimuli," in Electroencephalography and Clinical Neurophysiology, 1973, 34, pp 97–99:
The author describes a system allowing generation and presentation of modulated light stimuli with variable frequencies and wave forms. He concludes the possibilities of stimulation and positive responses during sleep-preparation and insomnia troubles.

o o o

Dr. William Harris, Director of the Penwell Foundation, USA in 1990:
Preliminary studies with audio-visual brain stimulators used by patients with AIDS indicate that "the devices are extremely efficient in terms of providing mental clarity, improved sleeping patterns (for sleep preparation and sleep duration) allowing for better physical disintoxication by the liver. The apparatus also stimulates immunology functions through states of deep relaxation."

o o o

Dr. Olivier Carreau, Saint-Louis Hospital in Paris, on "Efficiency of the MindsEye Plus audio-visual stimulator in treatment of the psoriasis during puvatherapy," study completed in January 1991.
Dr. Carreau analyzed 20 patients over a period of five months. Patients were treated one per week alternately via UVA and audio-visual stimulation (30-minute sessions) for psychosomatic skin disorders. All patients experienced deep relaxation during the sessions and had a feeling of well-being during the entire day. Five patients claimed that this feeling lasted for the following 2–3 days. Patients with combined therapy did better than with puvatherapy alone.

Transform Your iPod or any Android Player into a Portable Achievement Device

Find Out What You Can Achieve When You Dare to Relax!

Q MindFit + Your Brain = Success!

The Q MindFit delivers gentle pulses of light and sound combined with guided visualization and soothing music to take you to the profound levels of relaxation known for focus, learning, achievement, and healing.

Want to lose weight? Just click on one of 52 titles, then relax and let your mind do the rest.

Is playing better golf your thing? Any of more than a dozen visualization sessions can easily help you master the game.

Maybe you just want a little time to get away from life's stresses. No problem. Simply choose a program from the stress-free series and enjoy a mental vacation.

A 20 minute Q MindFit session can be equal to four hours of sleep. With hundreds of programs to choose from at Self-MasteryTechnology.com, there's simply no limit to how good you can feel and what you can achieve.

If you want to get more done in less time, Q MindFit is for you!

Your Q MindFit comes with everything you need—you simply plug your Q MindFit into the earphone jack of your iPod or Android player and you're ready to dream big!

Plus, when you register your Q MindFit, you get your own personal webpage for downloading new processes, tracking your progress and receiving updates.

There's no software to install. You can take your portable achievement device with you wherever you go

Self-Mastery Technology

If You're Ready to Transform Your Life from the Inside Out, You've Come to the Right Place...

Four Mind Technologies in One Mind-Blowing Pair of Glasses!
Light Frequencies Distinctive flashing light patterns train your brain to operate in the best possible mode for creativity, focus, and mindfulness. If you are the type who likes to get things done, this form of brainwave entrainment can transform you into a mental powerhouse with the right mindset, energy and clarity to accomplish just about anything.

Binaural Beats Put simply, these are imbedded tones that the brain naturally follows into states of deep relaxation. Within minutes your brain reaches extraordinary levels of performance that would otherwise take years of practice to achieve.

Self-Mastery technology (SMT) can help you change the way you view yourself and your life. Once you have a new image of yourself—as a healthy, happy, optimistic person—your fears and frustrations fade away and you no longer let small things stress you. SMT makes sure you are focusing on everything you want out of life so you can have it, effortlessly!

Mind-Music The music you hear on every PorterVision process is designed to create a full 360 degree experience that floods your mind with beautiful images and peaceful thoughts.
And so much more!

With Q MindFit You'll Enjoy all these Benefits and More!

- The relaxation response replaces the fight-or-flight response.
- The right and left hemispheres of the brain become more balanced.
- Blood flow to the brain increases, resulting in clearer thinking, better concentration, improved memory, and enhanced creativity.
- Serotonin levels increase, calming the mind and body and creating an overall sense of well-being.*
- Endorphin levels increase, providing the brain with alertness, acting as a natural anti-depressant, providing relief from pain, and creating pleasurable and loving feelings.*
- Because 20 minutes on the Q MindFit can be like getting four hours of sleep, you'll find yourself sleeping less, feeling more rested, and accomplishing more.*
- Energy levels soar.
- Relationships become more fulfilling.
- Career satisfaction improves.
- A sense of purpose develops.
- The ability to make personal changes, such as losing weight, quitting smoking, ending nail biting or other nervous habits happens faster and easier.
- And last, but certainly not least, one gains a seemingly effortless ability to handle and manage stress.

Most people would pay thousands of dollars for a magic pill that offers these kinds of benefits. By using the Q MindFit, you see results in just a few relaxing minutes a day!

Books Featuring Q MindFit Technology

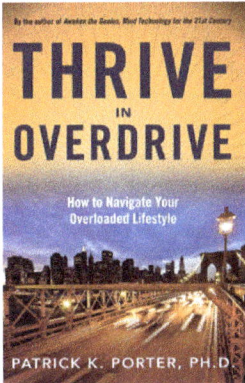

Thrive in Overdrive
How to Navigate Your Overloaded Lifestyle
Patrick K. Porter, Ph.D.

In today's high-tech, fast-paced world, no one is immune to stress. Why? Because our lives are too overloaded. Thrive in Overdrive shows you how to rid yourself of the happiness-robbing condition called stress and enjoy a balanced life, but without giving up your overdrive lifestyle that makes sure you stay ahead of the game. The book, written by recognized how-to self-help expert, Dr. Patrick Porter, is based on methods that have been time-tested by over a million clients worldwide. He uses true stories, anecdotes, and deceivingly simple creative visualization exercises to demonstrate that, yes, you can have it all.

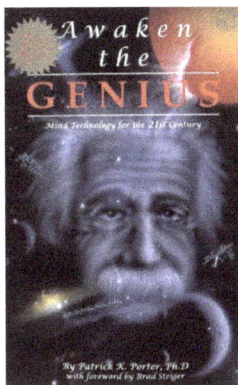

Awaken the GeniusMind Technology for the 21st Century
Patrick K. Porter, Ph.D.

You'll discover how to maintain a Genuine positive attitude...how to unleash your personal passion and Enthusiasm (including stories and fun-to-do exercises)...how to develop Non-stop energy and center that energy on reaching your goals...how to activate your unlimited imagination and creativity...how to enjoy and unending drive to succeed...and...how to experience every day what geniuses throughout history have enjoyed-spontaneous intuitive breakthroughs.

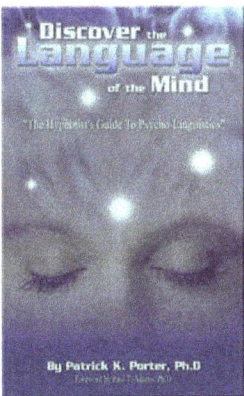

Discover the Language of the Mind
Patrick K. Porter, Ph.D.

Discover the Language of the Mind, the Hypnotist's Guide to Psycho-Linguistics was previously published as Psycho-Linguistics, The Language of the Mind. This fully revised edition includes updates on dozens of new developments in the hypnosis field, full transcripts for each of the eleven processes, which includes two never-before published techniques as developed and tested by Dr. Patrick Porter. Psycho-Linguistics is a practical guide to the combined theories of hypnosis, Neuro-Linguistic Programming, Creative Visualization and Accelerated Learning - a perfect 'mind guide' for experienced hypnotists and psychotherapists or for anyone seeking a quick, easy, step-by-step method for self-improvement and enhanced communication.

Six Secrets of G. E. N. I. U. S.
Patrick K. Porter, Ph.D.
Cynthia J. Porter, Ph.D.

Discover what inventors, artists and other great minds have known for centuries-the secrets of sparking their own creativity and super-charging their motivation. Learn simple strategies to rid yourself of negative thinking...to awaken your positive attitude in every situation...and to think your way through complex or confusing challenges. Discover what inventors, artists and other great minds have known for centuries-the secrets of sparking their own creativity and super-charging their motivation. Learn simple strategies to rid yourself of negative thinking...to awaken your positive attitude in every situation...and to think your way through complex or confusing challenges.

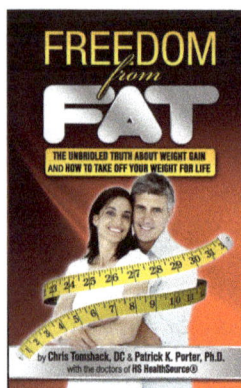

Freedom From Fat
The Unbridled Truth about Weight Gain
and How to Take off Your Weight for Life

Patrick K. Porter, Ph.D.

Chris Tomshack, DC

And the Doctors at HealthSource® Chiropractctic

This is not another diet book! Rather, it's your chance to finally understand why you're gaining weight and how to reverse the cycle. By following the advice of these doctors, you can achieve safe, healthy and lasting weight loss success. If you're looking for a real world, step-by-step plan for taking off your weight and keeping it off, brought to you by doctors who are helping patients succeed even when all else has failed, this book is your answer.

Within these pages you will discover:

- *Why fad diets, gimmicks and complicated diet plans are doomed from the start*
- *The underlying condition that makes it nearly impossible for some people to lose weight, and how to fix it*
- *A system that addresses every part of the weight puzzle-diet, mental attitude, habits*
- *How to change the core causes of cravings, conditioned overeating, and weight gain so you can keep your weight off for life*

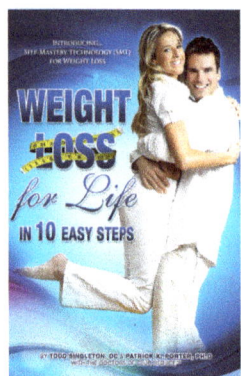

Weight Loss For Life in 10 Easy Steps

Todd Singelton, DC

Patrick K. Porter, Ph.D.

If you could lose weight on your own, you wouldn't be holding this book in your hands right now. The experts all tell you to eat fewer calories and exercise more. If only it were that easy! The truth is, most people and most so-called experts have no idea what triggers the body to gain or lose weight. Few people recognize the clues (symptoms) that are your body's warning signals that your food choices aren't working. Add the fact that almost no one understands the relationship between stress and weight, and it's no wonder we have a nation of chronic dieters who stay overweight, unhealthy and unhappy no matter how hard they try. Well, today is your day...because you have in your hands the definitive guidebook for weight loss success that lasts. Within these pages we'll teach you everything you need to know to lose weight and keep it off for life, and it couldn't be simpler when all you have to do is follow ten easy steps! Together, we'll finally make your dream a reality so you can...

- Stop starving
- Be rid of cravings
- End emotional eating
- Turn off fat storage hormones
- Supercharge fat burning hormones
- Suppress your appetite naturally
- Clear up digestive problems
- Reverse the stress/weight effect
- Do away with habitual overeating
- Achieve radiant good health from the inside out!.

Welcome to The Gift of Love Project

The Gift of Love is a poetic writing that has its own beauty … and upon further examination, it may lead one to a contemplative process, creating balance and harmony in one's everyday life. Over time, this process can also create subtle positive change in the recipient of The Gift.

My guidance leads me to distribute this writing to one billion people within the next two years. Hopefully, many people will be led to practice the contemplative process. If The Gift of Love resonates with you, please share it with others. As we gather and hold the power of love in our consciousness, we will dramatically reduce the level of anger, fear, and hatred on our planet today. -- Jerry DeShazo

The Gift of Love

I Agree Today
To Be The Gift of Love.

I Agree to Feel Deeply
Love for Others
Independent of Anything
They Are Expressing,
Saying, Doing, or Being.

I Agree to Allow Love
As I Know It
To Embrace My Whole Body
And Then to Just Send It
To Them Silently and Secretly.

I Agree to Feel it, Accept it, Breathe It
Into Every Cell of My Body on Each In-Breath
And On Each Out-Breath
Exhale Any Feeling Unlike Love.

I Will Repeat This Breathing Process Multiple Times
Until I Feel it Fully and Completely
Then Consciously Amplify In Me
The Feeling of Love and Project It to Others
As The Gift of Love.

This is My Secret Agreement –
No One Else Is To Know it.

For more about The Gift of Love Project and to view the videos, please visit www. TheGiftofLove.com. You will also be given access to a special 9-minute Creative Visualization that will align you with the Power of Love and supercharge your day. Together we will change the world one person at a time.

http://www.thegiftoflove.com/

ISBN: 978-1-937111-31-1

Printed in the United States of America

QMindFit